DISEASES AND PARASITES OF CATTLE

Editor
Gove Hambidge

BIOTECH
2019
Biotech Books
New Delhi - 110 002

Original Title: Livestock Yearbook of Agriculture, 1942

ISBN 978-81-7622-085-9

Published by : **BIOTECH BOOKS**
4762-63/23, Ansari Road, Darya Ganj,
New Delhi - 110 002
Ph.: 011 43003222
e-mail: biotechbooks@yahoo.co.in

Laser Typesetting : **Classic Computer Services**
Delhi - 110 035

Printed at : **Chawla Offset Printers**
Delhi - 110 052

PRINTED IN INDIA

CONTENTS

INTRODUCTION

Brucellosis of Cattle

Abortion, sterility and diminished milk and meat production are among the train of evils that follow infection of cattle with the *Brucella abortus* germ, the cause of brucellosis or Bang's disease. The losses due to this disease have been estimated very conservatively at $30,000,000 a year. It is introduced into healthy herds primarily by the addition of infected cows or infected pregnant heifers. The germ also causes undulant fever in human beings, but this danger can be greatly reduced by pasteurizing milk and by taking precautions in handling infected animals. Brucellosis cannot readily be diagnosed by the symptoms alone, but a blood-agglutination test, properly carried out; is a dependable means of diagnosis.

Lash and O'Rear point out that livestock owners spend large sums of money every year for remedies for abortion caused by bovine brucellosis and they mention careful experiments conducted by the Department of Agriculture with two of those remedies, which proved that they were absolutely worthless.

In 1934 a brucellosis control and eradication project was begun in connection with the cattle-reduction programme necessitated by the drought of that year. It was then estimated that 10 percent of the cattle in the United States were infected with the disease–twice the percentage that were infected with tuberculosis in 1917, when the tuberculosis eradication programme began. The brucellosis programme called for testing all dairy and breeding cattle over 6 months of age. At first begun with scattered herds, it was subsequently changed to an area basis in many States. Cattle owners are partially reimbursed for the slaughter of animals that react positively to the test. Re-tests are applied at frequent intervals and owners are carefully instructed as to the sanitary measures necessary to eliminate the disease. Many counties have now been certified as practically free of bovine brucellosis. Cattle owners participating in the programme have reported excellent results in increased calf crops, reduced sterility, higher milk production, lower costs and improved sales of breeding stock.

Meanwhile extensive field trials of calfhood vaccination against brucellosis were going on and these were so successful that since December 1940 almost all the States have adopted a vaccination programme as part of the general control project. In this programme, vaccinated animals gradually replace positive reactors.

Another method used effectively to supplement test-and-slaughter or vaccination is sanitary control. In herds where this method is adopted, animals about to calve or abort are placed in an isolated maternity barn, shed or stall and special sanitary precautions are observed in handling them.

General preventive measures in the fight against bovine brucellosis include such practices as adding only tested or accredited stock to the herd, segregation and testing of each animal added, testing of animals that have been sent to fairs or shows, diversion of drainage from infected premises, proper pasturization of milk used for feeding and precautions against introducing infection on clothing.

Johne's Disease

A gradual wasting away and an intermittent, increasingly severe diarrhoea are the chief visible symptoms of Johne's disease or para-tuberculosis, which affects cattle chiefly but also sheep, goats, deer and horses. As Simms, Mohler and Johnson point out, symptoms take a long time, months or even years, to develop and sometimes an animal can have a severe case yet show no apparent symptoms. The disease is incurable and fatal. It is caused by a bacillus very much like the tuberculosis organism and spreads by direct contact or through contaminated surroundings. There is reason to believe that it is much more prevalent in the United States than has been realized and it may also be increasing; a recent test of some 5,000 cattle in the Southeast showed positive reactions in 1 out of every 10. A positive johnin test (much like the tuberculin test) is considered to indicate the disease, though not all animals with the disease react positively to the test.

When Johne's disease appears in a herd, the owner faces at least a 2-year fight to get rid of it and unless he gets rid of it, it is likely to ruin the herd. A programme of control, as outlined by these authors, includes frequent, regular testing, removal of all reactors, thorough disinfection measures and strict sanitary precautions. In several States, indemnities can be paid for the slaughter of cattle with Johne's disease on the same basis as for the slaughter of tuberculous cattle. Since human beings are not subject to the disease and it does not damage edible parts of the carcass, the meat is suitable for human consumption, subject, of course, to inspection.

There are uncertainties and difficulties about this insidious disease that make it impossible to say as yet that its conquest is clearly in sight. For that, additional facts need to be uncovered by research.

Bovine Mastitis

It is not unusual to find infectious mastitis in half the cows in many dairy herds. The total annual loss that results from reduced production, poor quality milk and seriously diseased cows is enormous. There are two forms of mastitis–chronic and acute. The disease usually occurs in the chronic form and is difficult to detect. The acute form, which is a flare-up of the chronic form in most cases, is easily recognised by redness and swelling of the affected quarter, reduced milk flow and marked changes in the appearance of the secretion. In advanced cases of chronic mastitis, the quarter becomes hardened and milk production is greatly reduced. The disease is caused by bacteria, which are spread on the hands of milkers or in the cups of milking machines.

The best method of controlling the spread of mastitis is to segregate the infected animals and use sanitary measures. Detection of diseased cows and supervision of the control programme should be entrusted to the veterinarian. When the infected animals have been separated from the healthy ones, the producer can detect mastitis in its early stages in the latter group by the regular use of the strip cup and the btomthymol-blue test.

In the control programme, healthy cows are milked before the infected ones at every milking. Strict sanitary procedures, outlined by Miller, are additional safeguards to prevent spreading of infection. A grain ration high in protein should be avoided. Everything possible should be done to protect the udders from injury.

Blackleg

Blackleg, one of the really deadly diseases of cattle, affects mostly young animals 6 to 18 months of age. The organism that causes it enters the body through small wounds in the skin or the mucous membranes of the mouth and quickly causes extreme symptoms, including rapidly swelling tumors, high fever, great depression and violent convulsions. Death usually occurs with in 36 hours and the carcass rapidly becomes bloated by gas.

There is no cure for blackleg, but Mohler points out that five kinds of vaccine have been developed, anyone of which will make animals immune for 12 to 18 months, the period depending on the vaccine used. There is also an antiblackleg serum for treating calves already affected, but it cannot be relied upon to stop the progress of the disease.

When an animal has died of blackleg, the carcass should at once be completely burned or deeply buried and covered with quicklime. Any place when the animal has lain should be disinfected with a strong disinfectant. Since the organism is very resistant to destruction and may linger in pastures for a long time, annual vaccination is the only way to conquer the disease.

Shipping Fever or Hemorrhagic Septicemia

Hemorrhagic septicemia, as the name implies, is a poisoning of the blood (often quickly fatal), accompanied by internal hemorrhages. It has been considered that a specific germ, *Pasteurella boviseptica*, causes the disease, but some authorities now believe that, as in the case of swine influenza, it is the result of the combined action of a germ and a virus. In the main it attacks young cattle, especially those in poor condition that have been exposed to severe shipping conditions–lack of rest and proper shelter, irregular feeding and watering, etc.–during bad weather. The symptoms, described by Stein, are often severe and a fatal pneumonia is a rather common complication. Since the disease is infectious, the carcasses of animals that have died of it should be safely disposed of and the premises should be thoroughly disinfected.

Primary emphasis in preventing hemorrhagic septicemia must be placed on proper shipping of animals, including ample provision for feed, water and rest to conserve their vitality and the following of simple precautions with animals that have just been received after shipment. In many instances, if the injections are administered at the proper time, good results follow injection with a bacterian or aggressin, which produces a lengthy immunity or of an antiserum, which quickly produces a brief immunity and has some curative value. The use of these products, as well as the treatment and diagnosis of the, disease, should be left to a competent veterinarian. Diagnosis is often difficult because various other diseases have similar symptoms and laboratory tests may be necessary.

Milk Fever

Among the serious maladies of dairy cows, says Giltner, milk fever is the most common; moreover, it affects the high-producing cow rather than the poor one and usually strikes during the best part of her life. The disease commonly occurs soon after calving, the first symptom being a general depression, followed by nervousness and spasms, then collapse and finally loss of consciousness. Untreated animals are likely to die very soon.

At first thought to be due to infection of the udder, the disease is now considered to be caused or at any rate it is always accompanied, by a marked shortage of calcium in the blood, together with an unbalanced condition of other minerals. Treatment, which is highly successful unless there are complications with other diseases, consists in injecting calcium gluconate into the veins, or, with extreme sanitary precautions, inflating the udder with filtered air. An animal in a state of collapse should be kept from lying on its side as there is grave, danger that regurgitated material will get into the lungs and cause pneumonia.

No positive methods of preventing milk fever are known and those that might be helpful are accompanied by certain other dangers. A special ration before and at the time of calving is a wise precaution.

Miscellaneous Diseases of Cattle

In this article, Knudson and Creech give a concise account of a number of cattle diseases, with particular attention to symptoms and possible measures for prevention and control.

White scours (infectious diarrhoea or acute dysentery)

A contagious and infectious disease of young and newborn calves, caused by micro-organisms; particularly colon bacilli, which enter the digestive tract by way of the navel cord at birth or the mouth later on. Chief symptom, a profuse light-coloured diarrhoea with a characteristic odor; also weakness, lassitude and other signs of a general disturbance. Severe attacks may be fatal. Diagnosis is often difficult, since diarrhoea may be due to various other causes. Medicines are of little use after symptoms appear; inoculation with hyperimmune calf-scour serum soon after birth, before any infection takes place, will help prevent heavy losses. The chief aim should be to prevent infection of the newborn calf. Knudson describes the sanitary measures that should be taken before, at the time of and immediately after birth, including suitable disinfection and strict cleanliness. He also outlines a plan for the care and proper feeding of the very young calf from the time it takes its first feeding of colostrum milk and tells what to do if the disease appears.

Acetonemia (ketosis or chronic milk fever)

This disease of dairy cattle, particularly of heavy milkers, is discussed in the article on Nutritional Diseases of Cattle.

Pseudorabies (mad itch, infectious bulbar paralysis or Aujeszky's disease)

An infectious disease of cattle, not very common in the United States, caused by a virus which attacks the central nervous system (brain). Often rapidly fatal. Common symptoms, intense itching, drooling at the mouth, high temperature, weakness, paralysis. The disease affects hogs and is rather common among rats; both may be carriers and rats especially are suspected, though the actual mode of transmission is not definitely known. There is no known treatment. If the disease appears, the diseased animals should be isolated and their quarters thoroughly disinfected; hogs should not be permitted to run with the cattle; rats should be exterminated.

Papilloma or common warts

Several kinds of tumors affect cattle, but as Creech points out, most of them are rare. The most common are warts, cancer of the eye and internal tumors affecting the lymph glands. Common warts of cattle are infectious or catching and it has been proved that they are caused by a virus, which probably gains entrance through injuries in the skin. They may be large or small, appear almost anywhere on the body and spread to other areas. The chief damage is to hides, which are reduced in value. Creech describes treatment by tying off; clipping; surgery; the use of glacial acetic acid, silver nitrate and iodine and internal medication. A wart vaccine is now being used experimentally, with promising results. Prevention consists in removing warty cattle and taking suitable sanitary precautions.

Epithelioma (carcinoma or cancer eye)

A malignant tumor or cancer, affecting the eye or related tissues, but eventually spreading elsewhere in the body, with fatal results. Cause unknown; irritation and overe-xposure to strong sunlight may be contributing factors. There is no known cure after the disease has had a good start. Complete surgery of the cancerous tissue and the eyeball by a veterinarian usually gives satisfactory results if performed early enough. Otherwise, the animal should be sold for slaughter, subject to inspection.

Lymphocytoma (lymphatic leukemw or pseudoleukemia)

A cancerous, incurable, always fatal disease affecting the lymph glands primarily and showing various manifestations. The first noticeable symptom is usually an enlargement of the superficial lymph glands–submaxillary gland (throat), prescapular gland (shoulder), pre-crural gland (flank), supramammary gland (above the udder). Laboratory examinations may be necessary to distinguish the disease from tuberculosis and actinomycosis.

Actinomycosis and actinobacillosis

Chronic infectious diseases, the first caused by a fungus, the second by a bacillus, but both having similar symptoms. Actillomycosis causes enlargement of the bones of the head, particularly the lower jawbone (lumpy jaw), which become spongy and filled with pus. Actinobacillosis produces tumorous swelling and frequently ulceration of the soft tissues of the mouth and throat, often including the tongue (wooden tongue) and the lymph glands. Various internal organs may be affected. The mode of infection is not definitely known, but it is believed that the organisms gain entrance through injuries to the mucous membranes. Actinomycosis cannot be treated satisfactorily; affected animals should be fattened for slaughter. Actinobacillosis can be treated with suitable drugs and by surgery. There are special Federal meat-inspection regulations covering the disposal of carcasses of animals affected with these diseases, to which human beings are also susceptible.

Nasal granuloma (snoring disease)

A disease long known in India but only recently (1933) discovered in the United States and apparently confined to Louisiana. Chief symptoms, a thickening of the nasal mucus membrane, usually only the first 3 inches; many small nodules on the membrane; discharge of mucus, pus and sometimes blood from the nose; difficult breathing, accompanied by a snoring sound. The cause of the disease in this country has not been definitely determined; in India there are two forms, one caused by a parasitic worm, the other by a spore-bearing organism. Experimental treatments have so far not been successful.

Goiter

This disease is discussed elsewhere in this volume, under nutritional diseases. It is chiefly important in cattle as a disease of newborn animals due to iodine deficiency in the dam.

Specific Ophthalmia (infectious conjunctivitis, infectious keratitis or pinkeye)

Pinkeye usually begins as an inflammation of the conjunctiva (conjunctivitis), but may later involve the cornea (keratitis) and eventually destroy the sight. In addition to local redness, swelling, watering and discharge of pus, symptoms usually include Some fever, loss of appetite, decreased milk secretion and other signs of general disturbance of the system. The disease is believed to be infectious, with irritation or injury of the eye tissues as predisposing factor. Several organisms have been found to be associated with the condition, but it has not been proved that anyone of them is the specific cause. Healthy animals should be separated from those affected by the disease and the latter should be kept in dark stables or sheds, specially fed and dosed with Epsom salts. It is important to consult a veterinarian in cases of pinkeye to avoid serious results. Creech describes treatment with cocaine, silver nitrate, boric acid, mercurochrome and mixed keratitis bacterins.

Calf diphtheria

An acute, infectious, often fatal disease of sucking calves caused, by a widespread organism (*Actinomyces necrophorus*) which gains entrance through wounds in the mucous membrane of the mouth. Sometimes as many as 70 percent of the calves in a herd may be affected. The symptoms include extensive ulceration of the mouth caused by destruction of tissues, slobbering, a discharge from the nostrils, sometimes wheezing and coughing, depression, weakness and emaciation. Prevention consists in prompt isolation of sick animals and thorough cleansing and disinfection of quarters. Treatment, which is useful only in the early stages or in mild outbreaks, consists in removing dead tissue, painting ulcerated surfaces with appropriate medicinal agents, washing the mouth frequently with warm water and good nursing.

Pneumonia

An inflammation of the lungs caused by specific infections, parasitism (rarely in cattle), such conditions as chilling from exposure or foreign material getting into the lungs; often a secondary condition in some other disease. The symptoms may include dullness. Lack of appetite, high temperature, disturbed respiration, wheezing or, gurgling sounds in the lungs, diarrhoea, a discharge from the nostrils. Either death or recovery may be rapid or the disease may persist for several weeks. Treatment consists in good nursing, the use of tonics and stimulants, sometimes the application of counter irritants such as mustard plasters. There are no specific sera or vaccines such as are used for pneumonia in human beings, but large injections of blood from normal cattle are reported to be beneficial. Experiments with sulfonamide drugs have not progressed far enough to give definite recommendations. As Osteen points out, pneumonia demands treatment by a trained veterinarian.

Choke

Cattle do not chew thoroughly and food or foreign objects may lodge in the throat or lower down in the gullet, causing such symptoms as retching, coughing and eventually, bloating. If the object is in the neck, it may be possible to force it upwards by gentle manipulation with the hands. If it is in the chest region, it can sometimes be gently pushed downward to the rumen by the use of an oiled stomach tube fitted with a probang or slender wooden rod, at the end. If neither can be done, a veterinarian may have to operate. In any case, rough treatment should be carefully avoided. Before removing the object it may be necessary to relieve the pressure of gas by puncturing the abdomen with a trocar.

Cattle Coccidiosis

Coccidia, says Boughton, are minute parasites related to those that cause malaria. They multiply in the intestinal tract for a time, then change into oocyst–a resistant form–which are discharged in the feces and are picked up by cattle from contaminated surroundings. Practically all cattle become infected, not only once but repeatedly. Whether the infection is dangerous depends on the number of organisms taken in; small numbers may produce only mild symptoms or none at all. Cattle frequently recover spontaneously from attacks and many animals are carriers, constantly spreading infection though apparently not harmed themselves. Very young calves are especially susceptible to serious coccidiosis.

Among the symptoms of an acute attack are bloody diarrhoea, anemia, weakness and emaciation. Death may occur in a week or two, if it does not, the animal is likely to recover. Secondary complications, especially pneumonia, are common. There is no known medicine that will effect a cure, though the symptoms can be alleviated.

Boughton discusses in some detail the control methods that can be expected to prevent serious cases of coccidiosis. They include suck measures as daily removal of manure and contaminated bedding, careful sanitary precautions and isolation of young calves in individual box stalls if possible–if not, segregation of all calves in four age groups. Protection of young calves is the most important point later, the animals can usually withstand ordinary infections.

Cattle Tick Fever

A minute parasite called a piroplasm is responsible for cattle tick fever. The discovery that this parasite is carried by the cattle tick opened the way for a long series of discoveries regarding the means by which certain other diseases are transmitted–including such human maladies as malaria, fellow fever, Rocky Mountain spotted fever and typhus.

MacKellar tells how it also opened the way for a finish fight against this deadly disease of cattle, which used to be responsible for losses of 40 million dollars a year, not counting the indirect cost of burden- some restrictions and quarantines applied to the South.

In 1906 a campaign was begun to eradicate the tick–in itself a very damaging pest, quite aside from its role in spreading the fever. The method most commonly used in this campaign, which has been going on ever since, is to dip all the cattle in tick areas at regular intervals, usually every 2 weeks, during the tick season.

Gradually the ticks have been wiped out, until today the only places quarantined are a small area in Florida, where deer continue to harbor the ticks and another in Texas, where infestation filters in across the Mexican border. Losses from the disease are almost entirely eliminated and the removal of restrictions against former tick areas has been of immense benefit to the South.

The cost of the whole campaign to the Federal Government, the States and the counties has been little more than the former losses amounted to in a single year.

Anaplamosis: A Disease of Cattle

Anaplasmosis is known to exist in 23 of our own States and in many foreign countries. Characterized by marked anemia and depression, among other symptoms, this disease, caused by a minute parasite that invades the red blood cells, is fatal in 25 to 60 percent of the cases. Considerable research work, discussed by Stiles, has been done in recent years on the mode of transmission. It has been proved that the disease can be spread by the use of unclean instruments in such operations as dehorning, castration and the giving of injections, as well as by at least 18 species of ticks, 7 species of horseflies and several species of mosquitoes.

No preventive or cure has been discovered, but research is being carried on in this field. In some foreign countries., young animals are immunized by inoculation with the blood of a carrier, but these animals themselves become carriers, as does every animal that has recovered from the disease; hence the method is not used in the United States.

Because of the danger of spreading the disease through carriers, any animal that recovers should be fattened and sold for slaughter. Sick animals should be kept in the shade and given plenty of clean water, a little appetizing green feed, protection against insects and good nursing. Medicinal and other treatment by a veterinarian may include various procedures discussed by Stiles.

Cattle Scab and its Control

Four kinds of mites cause the contagious skin disease of cattle known as scab, mange or itch:

(1) Common scab caused by the psoroptic mite, which lives on the surface of the skin, was once a widespread menace in this country but is now rare as a result of a vigorous campaign of quarantine and eradication.

(2) Barn itch, caused by the sarcoptic mite, was once rare, but as Snyder points out, it has increased in the last few years and is now a very trouble some problem, Dairymen and breeders of purebred cattle can suffer heavy losses if the disease gets a foothold. The mites burrow into the skin instead of living on the surface and hence are more difficult to detect and combat than psoroptic mites.

(3) Chorioptic scab, caused by the chorioptic mite, is much like common scab but spreads slowly and is usually confined to the tailor legs.

(4) Follicular mange, caused by the demodectic mite, produces nodules or lumps on the skin that seriously damage the hides as leather, There is no practical remedy for this type of mange in cattle, but infected animals should be isolated.

The other three types of mange can all be controlled by dipping the animals in an officially approved solution of lime-sulfur or nicotine, For common scab and chorioptic scab, there should be two dippings10 to 12 days apart. For sarcoptic scab there should be four dippings at intervals of 6 to 10 days and just prior to the first one all affected areas on the body should be well scrubbed and soaked with the dipping solution. (One dipping of crude petroleum will kill this mite and apparently also the eggs, but it is injurious to the animals in some cases). In addition to dipping, all stables, enclosures and equipment that have been in contact with mangy cattle should be thoroughly cleaned and disinfected before being used for clean or dipped cattle.

Tapeworm and Roundworm Parasites of Cattle

The more important tapeworm and roundworm parasites of cattle take a heavy toll every year from the beef and dairy industries in the form of deaths from gross parasitism, lowered vitality, poor growth and production and the condemnation of meat and livers in packing plants. In discussing these parasites, Porter refers the reader to the article on sheep and goat parasites for further details, since the information in the latter field is more extensive and much of it applies to cattle.

Three groups of tapeworms are discussed:

(1) Those that live as adults in the intestines probably do less damage in cattle than in sheep., though calves may be sufficiently parasitized to be weak and unthrifty and hence should be excluded from pastures known to be a source of infection.

(2) Two tapeworms that infest dogs and other canines pass through an intermediate stage in cattle–the hydatid and the thin–necked bladder worm. To prevent infection, dogs on the place should be kept free of worms and stray dogs and wild canines should be kept off.

(3) A tapeworm of human beings occurs in the larval or bladder worm, form in the muscles of cattle, causing what is known as beef measles–oval white vesicles about the size of a pea. Proper sanitation prevents passing the infestation from human beings to cattle and thorough cooking of infected beef prevents passing it from cattle to human beings. Measly beef is condemned in federally inspected packing plants.

The roundworms included in the article are in five groups:

(1) Those infesting the lungs occur much more frequently in calves than in mature cattle. Heavy infestations cause progressive weakness and can prove fatal if the lungs are extensively involved, especially when a secondary bacterial invasion occurs. Infested animals should be removed from pasture to clean, sanitary quarters and given liberal quantities of feed.

(2) Three species of stomach worms infest cattle, producing such symptoms as gastritis, loss of flesh, general weakness, anemia and in some cases diarrhoea and bottle jaw. Calves and year lings are in general more seriously affected than adult animals.

(3) The small worms known as cooperids infest the small intestine chiefly and can cause extensive intestinal

inflammation calves, with diarrhoea, emaciation and anemia as symptoms in severe cases.

(4) The blood-sucking, cattle hookworm, a prevalent parasite of young animals, also causes emaciation, diarrhoea and anemia. The infective larvae, which can penetrate the skin as well as being swallowed, normally parasitize the small intestine.

(5) The nodular worm occurs in the large intestine and cecum, the attacks of the larvae producing nodules that are subject to bacterial invasion. Anemia, scouring and emaciation are among the symptoms in severe cases.

All the roundworms discussed are acquired largely from pasturage contaminated by droppings. Preventive measures include drainage of low wet areas (or excluding calves and yearlings from such areas), conservative stocking of pastures, rotation as often as possible, keeping calves away from older stock and from contaminated pastures and quarters, good sanitation and good feeding and isolation of infected animals for special treatment.

Medicinal treatment for cattle is much like that for sheep and in fact it is based largely on investigations with sheep. Worm medicines should be given only after competent veterinary diagnosis and advice; since their use is attended with danger to some of the animals. Porter discusses the use of some of the common anthelminthcs for parasites in the stomach and intestines.

Bovine General Trichomoniasis

Trichomonas foetus is a one-celled, microscopic, wriggling organism with three threadlike whips at the front end. When it infects effects the uterus of a cow, the result may be failure to conceive, abortion or death and disintegration of the fetus, though sometimes normal birth takes place. The disease is spread by infected bulls during service; but since it has been reported in virgin heifers, it may perhaps also be spread by close contact with infected cows. It was first reported in this country in 1932.

A tentative diagnosis can be made from the breeding history of the herd and of individual animals and a definite diagnosis by direct microscopic examination of material from the sex organs of the cow or bull or by culturing, the material.

There is no specific treatment for the disease. Cows that abort should be given a period of sexual rest. Generally no other treatment is required provided the abortion is complete. When the abortion is incomplete, that is, when part of the fetal membranes is retained and infection develops in the uterus, the case should be treated like any other form of uterine infection. Cows that fail to conceive should be allowed to pass two or three normal estrual periods without being bred. Cows that develop pyometra (pus in the uterus) should be treated by a veterinarian.

The use of infected bulls should be restricted to cows that have been exposed to the disease.

For prevention of the disease, Dikmans makes the following recommendations:

(1) Investigate breeding records before adding any animal to the herd or bringing any animal in or sending any animal away for breeding.

(2) Consult a veterinarian at once if breeding troubles occur; stop breeding operations temporarily if the trouble is due to trichomoniasis and determine which animals have been exposed to infection.

(3) Restrict the use of infected or suspected bulls that have had or have been exposed to the disease.

(4) Provide a new bull for heifers coming to breeding age and cows that have not been exposed.

Cattle Grubs or Heel Flies

The heel fly, warble fly or gadfly attaches its eggs neatly to separate hairs, mostly just above the hoofs of cattle. The fly itself does not sting or bite; it is unable to feed itself and lives only about a week. Its mere presence, however, terrorizes cattle much as some human beings are terrorized by snakes; during the heel fly season the animals lose flesh or fail to gain and milk production falls off. The eggs of the fly hatch in a few days and the grubs immediately burrow deep into the tissues, where they wander around, feeding and growing for about 9 months. Finally they reach the back and here each larva makes a hole in the skin and becomes enclosed in a pocket or cyst, remaining about 5 weeks and molting twice. Then it crawls out, drops to the ground and becomes a pupa. In 6 to 10 weeks the adult fly emerges. A female can lay as many as 300 eggs.

There are two species of heel flies, one confined to the North, the other common throughout the country. The fly season begins very early in the spring in the South and gradually spreads northward, terminating about the first of August at the northern limits of the flies' range. The damage done by the flies, as summarized by Laake, Bishopp and Wells, includes loss of production through nervous disturbance, the loss entailed in grub-infested meat, which has to be trimmed and discarded, injury to sausage-casing material and very extensive damage to hides. At the minimum, the losses due heel flies are estimated at 50 million dollars a year.

Much research has been done on methods of control. So far the best method seems to be to kill the grubs while they are in the backs of cattle. This may be done by applying derris or cube powder (5 percent rotenone) mixed with wettable sulfur. The material may be dusted on and rubbed in by hand or mixed with water and rubbed in with a stiff brush or sprayed on with a power sprayer. The last method is the most economical and the quickest for large numbers of animals, which are treated as they pass through a chute. The grubs may also be squeezed out of the backs of the animals by hand and extracted with forceps, a method that is slow but reputedly very effective in some cases.

The Stablefly

The big, vicious stablefly, which jabs painfully through the skin to suck its daily meal of blood, is a menace for three reasons, Bishopp and Laake point out–it worries and in large numbers can actually kill horses and cattle, it is an unbearable annoyance to human beings and it can carry infantile paralysis as well as such livestock diseases as hog cholera, anthrax and swamp fever. This last is the more serious because the stablefly can travel long distances; marked flies have been found to go as far as 52 miles.

The eggs are laid in moist, fermenting organic matter such as plant refuse or manure, in which the maggots live and grow; one female in a laboratory cage laid as many as 600 eggs. The most important single step in preventing infestations, then, is to eliminate such breeding places. For example, bale straw immediately without letting it get wet; scatter stack butts, grass clippings, vegetable trimmings and peanut litter immediately and manure at least twice a week instead of letting it pile up; spray windrows of beach grass with a mixture of creosote oil and fuel oil.

Where breeding cannot be entirely prevented, fly traps fitted in barn windows will catch some of the flies. Oil sprays containing rotenone or pyrethrum are even better. If the spray used on an animal contains as much as 10 percent of either of these extracts, it will give protection for a day or more.

The Horn Fly

Bruce estimates that in a herd of 500 head of cattle, with the common infestation of about 4,000 horn flies per animal (sometimes it runs much higher) the amount of blood extracted by the flies totals some 312 quarts in a year. In addition, these small, black, stabbing flies torment the animals, prevent them from eating properly and cause sores that may become infested with screwworms. The fly stays on the animal day and night, always resting with its head downward. It lays its eggs in droppings. Warm, damp, cloudy weather is especially favorable for the development of the insect.

The pest is harmful enough to warrant serious efforts to control it. In small pastures, the maggots may be killed by systematically scattering all droppings. Pyrethrum sprays can be used to kill the flies on the animals. A special fly trap, which Bruce describes, is also effective. It is a large boxlike affair through which the animal is forced to pass on its way to water or feed. An arrangement of curtains and weighted strips brushes the flies off its body; and the insects are caught in trapping elements as they try to get away. Some interesting tests have also been made in feeding cattle substances that would make the droppings poisonous to the fly maggots without harming the animals, but this work is still in the experimental stage.

Cattle Lice

Cattle in the United States are preyed on by the red louse, which bites, living on bits of skin and hair; two long-nosed blue lice; which suck blood; and the bloodsucking short-nosed ox louse. Infestation is worst during winter and spring, when the animals may sometimes be literally covered with lice and least in the hot weather of summer. The chief damage, Babcock and Cushing point out, is unthriftiness and lowered vitality; occasionally an animal succumbs to a severe attack.

Dipping in an insecticide is the best remedy and the best insecticide for this purpose consists of 100 pounds of wettable sulfur (325 mesh) plus 10 pounds of cube or derris containing not less than 5 percent of rotenone, to each 1,000 gallons of water. The animals are driven through the dipping vat, the head of each animal being ducked atleast once. Usually the first dipping is done in the early fall, followed by a second 12 to 14 days later and a third 17 to 21 days after the first dipping. If the third dipping must be omitted, two 17 to 21 days apart will give good control. Animals should not be hot when dipped and in cold weather they should be dipped early enough in the day to dry off before evening.

Coal-tar-creosote dips mixed in soft water are also effective. Arsenical dips are widely used but do not control the bull-nosed ox louse.

For a few animals only, the sulfur-rotenone mixture can be sprayed on with a bucket pump and rubbed into the skin by hand; or a dry mixture of 1 pound of the derris or cubs with 9 pounds of sulfur (325 mesh, wettable or non-wettable) may be dusted on and rubbed in. The dry powder should always be used in cold weather, especially in winter in the North. Second and third treatments should be given as in dipping.

Cattle Injuries Caused by Ingesting Foreign Objects

Giltner and Patton give photographs of an extraordinary collection of objects that have been recovered at various times from the stomach of cattle.

One of the fairly common results of swallowing a sharp object such as a nail or a piece of wire is that it eventually works its way forward to the heart sac, where it sets up an inflammation known as traumatic pericarditis that seriously affects the animal's general health and in the long run usually ends fatally. The symptoms of the condition and the post mortem findings are described by the authors.

Treatment is of little use, though in a few cases a radical surgical operation can be performed. Traumatic pericarditis and other injuries caused by ingesting foreign objects can be prevented, however, by keeping the premises free at all times of things that cattle might swallow–baling and barbed wire, for instance, staples, nails, scraps of metal. In many cases losses due to this cause have been eliminated by systematic clean-up and pick-up efforts.

Paint Poisoning in Cattle

Cattle are more sensitive to lead poisoning than any other

domestic animal, says Giltner and most cases are due to their licking. and swallowing lead paint. The danger exists on every farm; sometimes many animals in a herd are affected. Among the common early symptoms are slobbering, choking, colic, loss of appetite, reduced milk flow and constipation. The most striking symptoms, however–trembling, fits, apparent attacks of mania and blindness and deep coma-are caused by the effects of lead on the brain. Death occurs quickly in severe cases.

A few drugs are used by veterinarians to treat lead poisoning, but in most instances little can be done except to relieve the symptoms. The important thing is to prevent poisoning by seeing that the animals never have access to lead in any form. In particular, keep them away from freshly painted objects of any kind, see that paint cans are properly disposed of and use non-poisonous paints for objects from which cattle cannot be kept away, such as stalls and stanchions. In other words, always treat lead paint as a poison so far as cattle are concerned.

Nutritional Diseases of Cattle

In this review Madsen includes mineral deficiencies, vitamin deficiencies and certain miscellaneous disorders related to nutrition.

Calcium deficiency is rare in cattle, especially when they have roughage of good quality, but phosphorus deficiency is likely to occur when feed is restricted owing to drought, overgrazing or other causes or when feeds low in phosphorus make up a large part of the ration. The first apparent symptom is usually a depraved appetite; the animal chews bones and eats all kinds of material–some of it toxic–in an effort to get phosphorus. Later symptoms include loss of appetite, emaciation, weak bones, stiff joints, decreased productivity and reproductive failure. There are three ways to prevent or cure calcium or phosphorus deficiency–furnish feeds (listed by Madsen) that are good sources of these minerals, use mineral supplements or increase the mineral content and yield of forage by fertilising the soil. The author quotes figures on experiments with the feeding of a mineral mixture which show that this method can be a rapid and efficient means of increasing beef production on phosphorus-deficient range.

Recently an acute, sometimes fatal disease of high-producing dairy cows, common in the intermountain areas of the United States, has been found to be associated with a marked drop in the phosphorus content of the blood. Characterized by anemia and other blood abnormalities, general weakness, blood-tinged urine and other symptoms, it can apparently be prevented by liberal feeding of grain during the lactation period and regular use of a phosphorus-rich mineral supplement. Injections of dibasic sodium phosphate and drenches of this material or of bonemeal have been used successfully in treating the disease.

Calves fed rations low in magnesium develop acute symptoms characterized by temporary blindness and convulsions, as well as injuries to the blood vessels and heart. The trouble is not likely to occur unless the animals are fed too long on milk without supplementary feeds.

Grass tetany, a highly fatal disease of cattle recently turned out to good pasture, is characterized by a low blood content of magnesium and calcium, severe muscular spasms, violent cramps and paralysis. Treatment, if it can be given in time, consists in injecting calcium and magnesium chloride into the veins. Prevention consists in improving winter rations and regulating pasture feeding early in the season.

It is extremely important that cattle have an ample supply of salt. When the ration of dairy cattle is deficient in sodium chloride, there is a decline in condition and in milk yield and a loss of appetite, along with other symptoms.

Iodine deficiency is largely a sectional problem. When the dam is deficient in this element, her calf may be still-born or be weak at birth and die within a few days or it may be affected with a "big neck" (goiter) but appear normal otherwise.

"Salt sick" disease in Florida and "Grand Traverse" or "lake-shore" disease in Michigan have caused considerable losses among cattle in certain areas. A deficiency of cobalt or copper (and possibly iron and other minerals in some cases) is associated with these conditions, which may be identical and due primarily to anemia. In Michigan, cases have responded well to cobalt supplements in the ration; in Florida, a mineral mixture containing iron, copper and cobalt is recommended.

The selenium and fluorine problems are discussed in the article on Nutritional Diseases of Farm Animals.

So far as is now known, vitamin A and vitamin D are the only vitamins that must be supplied in the feed of cattle. A deficiency of vitamin A is by far the more likely of the two to occur and since it can be responsible for extensive losses, Madsen devotes considerable attention to it. Night blindness is one of the first symptoms that can be detected in adult animals, but, as the author points out, an animal may be getting enough vitamin A (or carotene) to prevent night blindness or other common symptoms and yet not nearly enough for normal reproduction and the birth of healthy calves. Calves severely deficient at birth are likely to have such symptoms as total blindness and convulsions and to survive only a short time. A watery swelling (anasarca) of the legs and forequarters characteristic of vitamin A deficiency has recently been observed in large numbers of fat cattle from the Corn Belt. The vitamin A problem should be in the forefront of the producer's planning of cattle rations, especially since animals may be critically low in this factor and yet appear to be in good condition.

Although many of the vitamins of the B complex are synthesized in the rumen of cattle, there is some evidence that the supply may not be sufficient to meet their needs under all circumstance–for example, in cases of infectious disease or intestinal parasitism. This point needs further research. Somewhat the same situation holds with vitamin C; recent work indicates that injections of this vitamin can in some cases markedly improve the breeding efficiency of both bulls and cows.

Evidence on the value of vitamin E in treating noninfectious barrenness in cattle in the United States is meager and conflicting.

Miscellaneous nutritional diseases discussed by Madsen include urinary calculi, bloat and ketosis. In the case of urinary calculi, many factors are suspected; those that are nutritional in nature include vitamin A deficiency and a lack of balance between calcium, phosphorus and magnesium intake. Bloat, a sporadic disease that often results in heavy losses, may be due, among other causes, to overeating or eating spoiled foods; Madsen discusses what is known about preventing and treating it, but points out that the problem needs further study. Ketosis, a disorder characterized by a high content of certain chemicals (ketone bodies) in the blood, urine and milk and a marked decline in milk flow, is an important problem in the dairy industry. Feeding corn sugar or molasses, increasing the grain allowance and improving the quality of the hay fed or putting the animals on good pasture will be beneficial in treating and preventing this condition.

Chapter 1

BRUCELLOSIS OF CATTLE

Elmer Lash & H.M. O'Rear[1]

[1] *Elmer Lash is Assistant Chief and H.M. O'Rear is Senior Veterinarian, Tuberculosis Eradication Division, Bureau of Animal Industry.*

The damage done to herds by brucellosis of cattle, the rapidity with which it spreads and the fact that the *Brucella* germ causes undulant fever in man make this disease especially important. A few years ago a Nation-wide campaign to eradicate it was begun; recently a new method of calfhood vaccination became a weapon in this campaign.

Brucellosis, an insidious disease commonly referred to as contagious abortion or Bang's disease, has caused heavy losses to the cattle industry every year, largely through reduced milk production, the loss of calves by premature birth and sterility. Brucellosis may spread very rapidly in a susceptible herd, many of the animals contracting the disease within a few weeks after they are exposed to the causative agent.

The disease is caused by a germ known as *Brucella abortus*, which is introduced into healthy herds by the addition of infected cows or infected pregnant heifers.

Brucella germs may be in the uterus or the udder of cows, in the generative organs of bulls, in certain lymph glands and joints and in the intestines and other organs of newly born calves. Diseased cows eliminate the germs in the fetus, afterbirth and uterine discharges for limited periods and in the milk for prolonged periods.

The malady appears to be commonly acquired through the mouth in feed and drink contaminated with the germs or by licking infected animals contaminated mangers or other objects to which the germs may adhere. The skin and the membranes lining the eyelids may also provide an entrance for the abortion germ. Proof that, bulls transmit the disease through the act of service is lacking.

It was not until 1896 that the organism responsible for bovine brucellosis was discovered by Professor Bang, noted Danish research worker. The existence of such a malady has been known for more than 100 years in the United States, however. For more than 40 years Department of Agriculture research workers have been continually engaged in investigations directed toward finding a cure or a means to control and eventually eradicate bovine brucellosis. Alice Evans, while an employee of the Department, did notable work in connection with brucellosis in discovering the similarity between the organism that causes abortion in cows and the corresponding organism in goats that causes undulant or Malta, fever in human beings.

Brucella Abortus and Human Health

In recent years it has been shown that undulant fever in man may be caused by the same germs that cause brucellosis in cattle, swine and goats. A large number of cases of undulant fever contracted from raw milk containing *Brucella abortus* have been reported. Handling infected pork products is also a means by which undulant fever is transmitted to man, as is the handling of discharges and aborted fetuses from infected animals. Though undulant fever would not be classed as a major health problem, it is nevertheless one to be reckoned with and it can be reduced materially through the eradication of the disease in cattle. Dairymen and breeders of meat animals are aware of the possibility that human beings may contract undulant fever from raw milk, meat and dairy products infected with brucellosis germs and of the influence this may have on the market for their products. The simple precautions of pasteurizing milk and cooking meat, however, make these foods safe for human consumption.

Symptoms of Brucellosis

The symptoms of brucellosis in cattle are rather inconstant and indefinite. Abortion is probably the most widely known and most readily observed symptom, but it may easily be misinterpreted, since not all cows that abort are affected with the disease. Moreover, the prompt recognition of the disease in affected herds is made more difficult by the fact that many animals that have it never abort. Sterility is usually a serious trouble in herds infected with *Brucella abortus*, but it does not constitute definite evidence of such infection. The retention of the afterbirth, likewise, does not definitely indicate the presence of the disease, as this condition, too, may occur when brucellosis is absent. None of these symptoms prove the presence or absence of the malady, but they may well be regarded as justifying suspicion and calling for prompt action. This is particularly true of abortion; until a definite diagnosis with the blood- agglutination test can be made, it is advisable to infer that an aborting animal is affected with the disease and to take action accordingly.

Diagnosis

In the blood stream of an animal infected with brucellosis there is an antibody, a substance known as agglutinin. When blood serum containing this substance is brought in contact with a suspension of *Brucella* organisms (called an antigen), it causes the organisms to adhere to one another and form clumps. This action, known as agglutination, is the basis for the test used in diagnosing brucellosis in the living animal.

To obtain the serum for a test, a sterile needle is inserted through a disinfected spot of skin into the jugular vein of the animal and a small amount of blood is drawn into a sterile test tube or small bottle. This is allowed to set for a few hours, until the serum separates from the blood clot. A carefully measured amount of the serum is then mixed with a carefully measured amount of antigen for the test. There are two methods of making the test, the tube method and the plate method and either one is remarkably accurate when conducted by an experienced operator.

Losses from Brucellosis

Although it is difficult to determine the financial losses caused by this insidious disease even approximately, estimates, based mostly on actual losses in various communities have varied from 30 million dollars annually to much larger amounts. No definite, detailed survey taking into account the tremendous intangible losses has yet been made and hence all estimates have probably fallen far short of the real situation. It is not enough to figure the probable value of a calf that is born dead or that is weak and soon dies, the shrinkage of beef in the beef animal, the diminished production of milk in the dairy animal, the temporary or permanent sterility that may follow the infection and not in frequently, the loss of the cow itself through infection; there is also the financial loss that the breeder of selected purebred cattle suffers from interference with his breeding programme because of the presence of the disease in his herd.

A careful study of a herd maintained at an experiment station showed that the loss per cow in milk production alone was over $100 a year. In another study it was determined that the loss resulting from abortion in a good commercial grade herd of 16 cows was about $135 annually and in a typical purebred herd, $486. Veterinarians and cattle breeders know the wide distribution and economic importance of brucellosis and the trouble it has caused them makes them more interested in it than in any other infectious disease of cattle. From general observation and special studies, it is known that at the time the cooperative State and Federal campaign to eradicate brucellosis was inaugurated in July 1934 the disease was more widespread than it had been some years before.

Remedies Worthless

There is no drug, chemical or medicinal compound that has been proved to be effective in the prevention or cure of brucellosis, but livestock owners of this country have spent large sums annually for worthless remedies in an effort to stop abortion in their cattle due to bovine brucellosis. These remedies have gained popularity because in most instances they are used and their value is judged at a time when the disease has run its course and is becoming chronic. At this stage abortions can be expected to decrease as a result of acquired immunity and a large percentage of the cows produce apparently normal calves. Perhaps no other disease is so deceptive in its apparent response to treatment as brucellosis. Though the Department had frequently warned the public that no drug or combination of drugs had been found to be effective in combating this malady in cattle, traffic in so-called cures continued for a time to flourish. It was decided therefore, in 1936, to conduct some experiments with two of the remedies that had been widely advertised. One hundred heifers were selected to be the subjects of the experiments, which were carefully controlled. The two products were proved to have no value whatever in preventing abortion or curing brucellosis in cattle.

Control and Eradication

Brucellosis of cattle may be controlled in several ways, the method used depending on herd conditions and the severity and extent of the disease in the herd. Four methods of control have been used successfully: Test and slaughter, calfhood vaccination with a culture of reduced virulence, sanitary control or herd management and test and segregation.

The Test and Slaughter Method

Since 1896 methods of control have been established, but unfortunately none of those thus far receiving recognition are easy of operation or inexpensive. Consequently, there was little organized effort to control the disease until July 1934, when funds were made available by Congress for a cattle-reduction programme associated with the severe drought of that year. Since such a programme was to be inaugurated, it seemed logical to direct it in part toward the elimination of diseased cattle and part of the funds were allotted for this purpose. Thus in July 1934 the present brucellosis control and eradication project was begun in cooperation with the livestock sanitary officials of the various States. Since then the cattle owner's losses have been gradually reduced and are now very much less than they were at that time.

The plan promulgated at the beginning of the campaign, when it was estimated that there were 10 million surplus cattle in the United States, called for subjecting all dairy and breeding cattle over 6 months of age to a blood-agglutination test. It also provided for the slaughter of the animals that reacted to the test, since it is accepted as a fact that such animals are affected with bovine brucellosis.

This was a huge undertaking. It was necessary to draw a sample of blood from each animal under supervision and forward the samples to a laboratory for test. A corps of technicians had to be trained to make the tests and in order to meet the emergency the laboratories of many of the States were expanded and new ones established. The Department purchased a number of trailer laboratories that have proved very satisfactory. They are usually set up in the county seat where cattle owners may see the blood of their animals being tested and thus gain a clearer understanding of the methods employed to detect diseased animals. High-school teachers and students are invited to view the work conducted in the trailer laboratories and this has proved very interesting as well as educational to the young people.

When work was inaugurated in the cooperative eradication of bovine brucellosis and until more cattle owners understood the advantages to be derived from a herd free from this disease, only scattered herds were tested. Then, as owners who had freed their herds of the malady realized that bovine brucellosis is easily spread from one farm to another, there were urgent requests to test all cattle in an area and destroy diseased animals that might serve as reservoirs of infection from which the disease might be carried back into the tested herds. Acting on these requests and requests from owners whose herds had not been tested, many of the States took up cooperative eradication work on an area basis.

The Area Plan

Under the area plan, all the cattle in an area, except steers and calves under 6 months of age, are tested and the reactors removed and slaughtered. Retests are applied at the proper intervals. The owners are given instructions as to the sanitary method to follow, since proper sanitation is a very important factor in eliminating the disease. In December 1939 the plan of designating areas as practically free of brucellosis was inaugurated. Whenever the tests of all cattle in a county 6 months of age and over, except steers, indicate that the percentage of cattle with positive reactions does not exceed 1 percent of those tested and that the number of infected herds does not exceed 5 percent of the total number, the regulations provide that such a county may be declared a "modified accredited Bang's disease-free area" for 3 years by the cooperating State and Federal officials in charge of the work, provided all infected herds are placed in quarantine. The cattle in these herds must be retested for the disease at intervals of 30 to 90 days until all of them pass two successive negative tests and they must also pass a third negative test not less than 6 months from the date of the second. The reactors in any test are of course removed from the herds and disposed of in accordance with the State and Federal regulations. On February 1, 1940, the first countries–209 in 17 States–were declared modified accredited areas in recognition of progress made in combating brucellosis. By November 1, 1941–almost 2 years later–the total of such counties had reached 446. They were located in 23 States and constituted 14.5 percent of all the counties in the United States.

Almost all the States also have provisions for accrediting individual herds of cattle as free from brucellosis.

In such areas brucellosis can be eradicated at relatively small cost and with very small loss to the cattle owners by continuing the testing programme and slaughtering the reactors. This is undoubtedly the quickest and most practical procedure except in the badly infected herds in such areas in which infection persists after several tests have been made.

Indemnity Payments and Progress

The cooperative programme inaugurated in July 1934 provides for partially reimbursing cattle owners for animals slaughtered as reactors to the test for brucellosis. During the first few years of the campaign the Federal Government provided a major part of the indemnity payments. Since May 1, 1939, however, the Bureau of Animal Industry has been forbidden by Federal statute to make indemnity payments to owners for the slaughter of reactors unless the State or municipality pays a sum equal to or greater than that paid by the Bureau. Federal payment is made on the basis of one-third of the difference between the appraised value and the salvage value, but this amount is not to exceed the amount paid by the State and it is not to exceed $25 for a grade and $50 for a purebred animal.

During the first 7 years in which this project was conducted, agglutination blood tests, Including retests, were applied to approximately 48,117,000 cattle and disclosed about 2,134,000 reactors. At the end of the 7-year period, approximately 1,184,000 herds, containing about 13,933,000 cattle, were under supervision throughout the United States for the control and eradication of brucellosis. About 1,175,000 cattle were in the herds of cattlemen who had applied for the test and were on the waiting list.

Benefits of the Campaign

During the, progress of the cooperative control and eradication campaign the Bureau of Animal Industry has received numerous reports of benefits derived from the programme. Typical benefits reported by participating cattle owners include thriftier condition of herds; calf crops, in both beef and dairy herds, approximately 20 to 25 percent greater than formerly; noticeable decreases in the number of cows affected with udder troubles and sterility; and material increases in the milk production of herds, roughly comparable to the number of diseased cows replaced by healthy ones. The following report interestingly illustrates this last point. In the first test, applied to 8,304 cattle, 2,319 reactors were reported or an infection at the rate of 27.9 percent. Four years later the test of 7,403 cattle in the same area disclosed 59 reactors or 0.8 percent infected. The milk report of this area showed that 7,403 cows were producing 1,430 gallons more milk a day than the 8,304 cows did when brucellosis infection was active. The benefit to the dairymen is reflected not only in increased milk production but also in lowered operation and maintenance costs. Among additional benefits reported by cattle owners are greater marketability of breeding stock and better prices, because purchasers are becoming more and more insistent on disease-free sources of animals and State legislation is restricting the entry of untested breeding stock; greater marketability of dairy products, because legal restrictions are imposed by States, cities and towns on products from untested herds; and greater safety to human health, because raw milk from herds infected with brucellosis may transmit undulant fever.

Calfhood Vaccination

For a number of years studies have been in progress on a rather large scale for the purpose of determining the possibilities of a comparatively safe method of preventive vaccination with a vaccine developed in the laboratories of the Bureau of Animal Industry from a culture of the *Brucella* organism of low virulence.

This vaccine has also been subjected to rigid tests by many research workers in other similar institutions, with encouraging results. For many years the livestock interests and livestock sanitary officials alike have shared the hope that eventually some satisfactory means of artificially immunizing cattle against this malady might be perfected. Because brucellosis, particularly in dairy cattle, has a tremendous economic importance in addition to its human or public health significance, the prospect of another practical weapon in the control of this disease is of particular significance.

Field Trials

In addition to the information gained in studies of the vaccine, which; in the main, were conducted under the usual procedure employed in controlled experiments, it was decided to determine the effectiveness of calfhood vaccination under natural field conditions. A field project was started in January 1936 to determine the value of the vaccine when applied to calves under natural conditions and the feasibility of a vaccinating procedure as a practical means of controlling brucellosis.

Since the project was to be conducted cooperatively in privately owned herds, the usual experimental procedure of maintaining control animals was omitted. The herds selected, therefore, were chosen from those in which the disease was shown by the blood-agglutination test to be present, in a sufficient number of animals to insure adequate exposure of the vaccinated animals to the disease and no herd containing less than 15 per cent of positive reactors was accepted. Finally, 260 herds, containing approximately 19,000 cattle, were selected in 24 States. In the initial test applied to these herds, 29.2 percent of positive reactors and 8.4 percent of suspicious animals were disclosed. The suspects and reactors were retained in each herd for a time, after which the practice was adopted of eliminating a few each year as the vaccinated animals came into production and could serve as replacements. The vaccinated animals were permitted to mingle constantly with the infected members of the herd and the usual sanitary practices employed in animal disease control were not applied in these herds. The only means of control employed was the vaccination of calves between 5 and 7 months of age with *Brucella abortus* vaccine strain 19.

A summary of the results during the first 4½ years of the study, covering three pregnancies of the vaccinated animals, is as follows: In these herds 13,854 calves were vaccinated when between the ages of 5 and 7 months. There were 8,182 calvings of which 7,872 or 96.2 percent, were normal and only 310 or 3.8 percent, were abortions. Of the 310 animals that aborted, 182 or 58.7 percent, were negative to the test after calving and 1.28 or 41.3 percent, showed either a positive or a suspicious reaction. Consequently, on the basis of the blood-agglutination test, only 128 abortions or 1.6 percent of the 8,182 calvings, could be attributed to brucellosis. Of the 1,346 animals that calved normally and showed either a positive or a suspicious reaction to the test after calving, approximately 500 or 37.1 percent, were negative on the first retest applied 6 months later. Of the first group of 97 animals that calved normally during the first pregnancy and gave a suspicious or positive reaction to the test after calving, 75 or 77.3 percent, had returned to a negative reaction on the fifth retest, applied 2½ years later.

The results of the field trials as well as those of experiments with calfhood vaccination with *Brucella abortus* strain 19 showed that this method of control is very effective as far as calf production is concerned and markedly effective in actually preventing infection. Accordingly, the results of the field study were presented to the United States Live Stock Sanitary Association during its annual meeting in Chicago in December 1940 and a general plan for the official recognition of calfhood vaccination as an aid in cooperative brucellosis control was proposed by the Chief of the Bureau of Animal Industry. According to the provisions of the plan, calfhood vaccination, as well as the test-and-slaughter method of eradication, may be used in States where the proper officials deem conditions favorable, dependent on acceptance of the plan by the proper authorities in such States. Many of the States have adopted plans for using calfhood vaccination in the control of brucellosis in cattle and interested cattle owners should consult their State veterinarian or State livestock sanitary officials before having the vaccine used in their herds.

The aim in the use of vaccine in a brucellosis infected herd should be directed toward the eradication of the disease rather than merely toward the assurance of a calf crop. The eradication of the disease is possible only through the removal of the animals that continue to show an agglutination reaction on repeated tests. The reacting animals may be removed immediately, if necessary or gradually as vaccinated replacements become available. It should be obvious, therefore, that two things are necessary in this connection:

(1) That vaccination should be confined to calves between 4 and 8 months of age, and

(2) That periodic blood tests should be made of the entire herd. To obtain the desired results, the administration of the vaccine and subsequent care of the affected herd should be entrusted to a qualified veterinarian.

Sanitary Control or Herd Management

Another plan of control that is both practical and economical should not be overlooked. This is the sanitary control method, with special relation to herd management, which, though it involves extra work, pays splendid dividends. In many herds the disease has been controlled by this method, which has two requirements:

(1) A maternity barn, shed or stall sufficiently removed from buildings housing the other cattle to prevent direct exposure to infection and (2) A close, daily observation of each pregnant animal, especially first-term heifers. At the first indication of approaching calving or signs of abortion, the animal should be placed in the maternity barn and kept from the remainder of the herd until abortion or calving has occurred and discharge has ceased. Persons caring for these animals should carefully wash their hands with soap and water and thoroughly disinfect their boots or shoes before leaving the building. Implements used for feeding and watering should not be used anywhere else. The aborted fetus and afterbirth should be burned or buried with quicklime. Additional sanitary treatment should be given to aborting animals before they are returned to the herd and they should not be bred for at least 3 months. These sanitary control measures, when used in conjunction with the test and slaughter method or vaccination, greatly increase the efficiency of the latter two through the removal of possibilities of exposure.

Test and Segregation Method

This method consists in segregating the reactors to the blood-agglutination test in a separate herd apart from the nonreactors. Separate premises are necessary for each group. Retests at frequent intervals are made of the nonreacting group in order that infection may be detected in the beginning stage and the reacting animals, if any, removed. Many valuable herds have been freed from infection by this method, but there are several reasons why it is not a desirable one:

(1) Only a few owners can provide facilities for two herds;

(2) It is usually some time before the reacting herd can be disposed of; and

(3) A single act of negligence in the care of the nonreacting herd may result in undoing several years effort.

Prevention

The old adage, "An ounce of prevention is worth a pound of cure," is sound advice in regard to brucellosis and no possibility of preventing infection from gaining entrance to a normal herd should be overlooked. Undoubtedly the chief way in which this disease is introduced into a herd is through replacements or additions, especially of pregnant heifers cows. All animals added to a herd should be negative to the agglutination test or be purchased from herds accredited as being free from brucellosis, an it is advisable to keep them from direct contact with the herd for a period of 3 months and not admit them to the herd until they react negatively to the test. Animals shown at fairs and livestock shows may be exposed to infection and it is advisable to test them several months after their return. Drainage from adjacent infected premises should be diverted, if possible and small sluggish streams flowing through and from premises known to be infected should be fenced off. The proper pasteurization of milk will make it safe for feeding. Stockmen should be careful in visiting farms where infectious diseases exist, as the germs may be brought home on shoes or clothing.

Chapter 2

JOHNE'S DISEASE

B.T. Simms, William M. Mohler & H.W. Johnson[1]

[1] *B.T. Simms is Director and H.W. Johnson is Associate Veterinarian. Regional Animal Disease Research Laboratory, Auburn, Ala. and William M. Mohler is Senior Veterinarian, Pathological Division, Bureau of Animal Industry.*

The world "Insidious" can truly be applied to Johne's disease. It creeps up unobserved, the symptoms are mild at first and the end is death. It is one of the most difficult of diseases to eradicate from a herd-and apparently it is increasing in the United States. The authors tell what is known and what is not known about it.

Johne's disease or paratuberculosis, is a chronic infection characterized principally by inflammation of the intestines, loss of condition and diarrhoea. It attacks cattle and sheep and has been reported in goats, deer and horses. So far as is known, man is not susceptible. The disease is very widespread, having been observed in practically every country where cattle are raised on a large scale. It occurs very frequently in districts such as western continental Europe and the British Isles, where intensive dairying is practiced.

While Johne's disease has been found in both beef and dairy cattle in every part of the United States, accurate figures showing its extent in this country are not available. Both tests of live cattle with johnin (a diagnostic agent similar to tuberculin, prepared from cultures of the causative bacillus) and examinations of slaughtered cattle at packing plants have indicated that the disease is much more prevalent than most veterinarians and livestock sanitary authorities have realized. About 5,000 head of cattle, most of which were in dairy herds, were tested recently in the Southeastern States and over 100 percent gave positive reactions.

There are very few records of the occurrence of the disease in sheep in the United States, but only a few investigators have examined sheep for the disease.

Cause of the Disease

The causative agent of Johne's disease is a bacillus named *Mycobacterium paratuberculosis*, which is usually found in scrapings from affected parts of the intestinal mucous membrane and in the mesenteric lymph glands.[2] This organism does not grow readily on the commonly used laboratory culture media. Even on media especially adapted to it, it grows very slowly when first isolated from the tissues of diseased animals; hence obtaining cultures is a difficult and laborious procedure. After growing on laboratory media for several generations, however, the organism becomes adapted to such media and grows fairly well. So far as is known, it does not multiply outside the body of a host animal.

Attempts at infecting laboratory animals have met with little success. If the organisms are suspended in oil and injected intraperitoneally (into the lining of the abdominal cavity) into guinea pigs, local lesions or tissue injuries, usually develop on the liver, spleen and omentum, but a progressive disease does not follow. The rabbit gives evenless response. The chicken appears to be somewhat more susceptible than the guinea pig, but shows little evidence of a progressive disease.

Mode of Infection

Since the Johne's disease organism lives in the mucous membrane of the intestines of infected cattle and sheep, large numbers may be present in the feces of diseased animals and it is generally believed that this is the principal source of infection. Exposure may come from direct contact between infected and

---

[2] *Mycobacterium paratuberoculosis* is aerobic, nonmotile, sporeless, and acid-fast.

susceptible animals or through the use by susceptible animals of pens, pastures, corrals or barns that have been contaminated by diseased cattle or sheep. A contaminated water supply may be a potent source of the disease.

It is very generally believed that young animals are more susceptible than mature ones and that the route of infection is through the digestive tract.

In most herds the disease spreads rather slowly. Even where Johne's disease has been known to be present for many years and there has been no segregation of the infected cattle, it is rather unusual to find as many as half the herd affected.

Several months to several years may pass following exposure before infected cattle show clinical symptoms. Many such animals carry large numbers of the Johne's disease organism in their intestines and may be potent in spreading the disease.

Symptoms

Symptoms of Johne's disease are seldom observed in cattle under 1 to 2 years of age; there are very few records of the disease in steers or in heifers before their first calves are born. Probably the ordeal of freshening makes the infected cow more susceptible to the ravages of paratuberculosis, for the clinical symptoms often appear for the first time within 2 to 5 or 6 weeks following calving.

The symptoms that are considered typical consist in gradual loss of flesh to the point of emaciation and intermittent diarrhoea be- coming gradually worse. In most instances the temperature remains practically normal. The appetite is usually fairly good until the disease is well advanced and there is little or no apparent disturbance of the respiratory, circulatory and urinary systems. During attacks of diarrhoea there is some increase in thirst. The decline in general condition is usually accompanied by a roughening of the coat and drying of the skin. Diarrhoea may not appear until the animal has lost considerable weight. The semi liquid or liquid feces are usually free from blood and in most instances do not have a very foul odor until the disease is well advanced. Large numbers of gas bubbles may appeal in the feces, but this is not very common. There may seem to be improvement, but it is usually very temporary. The tendency is for the attacks of diarrhoea to become more frequent and severe until death occurs.

Diagnosis

Diagnosis of Johne's disease has always been somewhat difficult. Many infected animals that may be active spreaders of the disease show no clinical symptoms. Even those exhibiting symptoms may be suspected of suffering from malnutrition, parasitism, chronic indigestion or chronic poisoning. Attempts at finding acid-fast organisms in either the feces or scrapings from the rectum are sometimes successful, but in many known cases results have been negative.

The use of diagnostic agents similar to tuberculin has given encouraging results. The materials used and the methods of injection have varied with different workers. Twort and Ingram prepared johnin in the same manner as tuberculin and injected it subcutaneously (under the skin). Hastings, Beach and Hadley used avian tuberculin subcutaneously and Hagan and Zeissig injected it intravenously (into the veins). The reactions from these injections are a rise in temperature and, in some animals, a general systemic upset.

Intradermic injections (into, not under the skill) of johnin in infected cattle have resulted in local reactions comparable to those seen in tuberculous cattle following the intradermic injection of tuberculin. The reactions appeared in 1 to 3 days and disappeared slowly, but the seventy-second hour after injection is apparently the best time to observe results. The minimal enlargement that is considered a reaction to johnin is smaller than that interpreted as a reaction in tuberculin testing and the swelling also tends to be somewhat more diffuse than that in tuberculin reactors. Observations indicate that the intradermic injection of johnin does not cause a physical break-down in infected animals.

Practically all workers agree that animals that react to any of the Johne's disease tests are, in a high percentage of the cases, infected. The weakness in diagnosis with the tests is that some infected animals fail to react.

Since the organism causing Johne's disease is similar to that causing tuberculosis, there has been much interest in the possibility that animals affected with one of these diseases might react to tests for the other. Some cattle that have given typical reactions when tested with tuberculin have shown the presence of Johne's disease instead of tuberculosis on post mortem examination. In some herds cattle with no visible lesions have repeatedly reacted to tuberculin over a period of years and it has been established that paratuberculosis is present in such reactors.

Treatment

No satisfactory method of treating cattle affected with Johne's disease has been found. Some animals respond temporarily to a change in feed and treatment with intestinal astringents soon after symptoms appear. Some veterinarians have recommended that animals showing clinical symptoms be taken off pasture and given dry, nutritious feed, while others state that an alleviation of symptoms is frequently observed if affected cattle are placed on good pasture. All agree that any improvement is soon followed by a recurrence of symptoms. Practically all cattle that develop clinical symptoms die within a period that varies between 1 month and 2 years. It is usually recommended, therefore, that animals showing symptoms of Johne's disease be sold for beef while they are still in good condition. Since the disease is not transmissible to man and the lesions do not involve any of the edible parts, the carcasses of affected cattle in good condition at the time of slaughter, if they show no indication of any other disease, are passed as wholesome food.

Post-mortem Findings

The pathology of Johne's disease is restricted to the digestive tract and adjacent lymphatic glands. Both the location and the type of the lesions vary somewhat in animals of different ages. In young calves the entire small intestine may be involved, while in mature animals the lesions are usually restricted to the ileum, cecum, colon and rectum. In calves the principal changes observed on autopsy are those accompanying acute congestion. There is redness and some swelling of the mucous membrane of the affected portion of the small intestine. In some cases only a small area is involved.

The changes found in mature cattle indicate a much more chronic disease. The lesions consist principally of a marked thickening of the affected mucous membrane, with some reddened patches and some enlargement of the adjacent lymph nodes. In severe cases of long standing the mucous membrane may be 2 to 5 times its normal thickness. The thickened portions lie in folds, as if the lining membrane were too large. There may be few or many reddened patches and they vary greatly in size and characteristics. Some are rather sharply outlined; others are diffuse. In some cases these changes involve the mucous membrane of almost the entire ileum, cecum, colon and rectum, while in others only a small area may be affected. In mature cattle, lesions are found most frequently in close proximity to the ileo-cecal valve. Smears made from the thickened and reddened areas may reveal typical slender, rod-shaped, acid-fast bacteria, usually occurring in nests or clumps.

In some infected animals the organisms are very plentiful, while in others they are very scarce. There seems to be little relation between the severity of the lesions and the number of bacteria found on smears from them. Neither is there any marked relationship between the severity of the symptoms and the extent of the lesions. Some of the most severe advanced cases may have very slight lesions.

The thickening and fold formation just described are not necessarily indicative of Johne's disease. Such changes have been found in the mucous membranes of the intestines of many cattle which had passed johnin tests and in which the paratuberculosis organisms could not be found. It has been impossible to differentiate by macroscopic examination of the tissues between the lesions in cattle free from Johne's disease and those in affected cattle.

In sheep there are even fewer changes than in cattle. Reacting sheep in which Johne's disease organisms have been demonstrated have had only a slight thickening or reddenning of the mucosa of the intestines. Lesions have not been found in any other organs of sheep.

Control and Eradication

Since there is no known method of treating Johne's disease successfully, any effective control must consist in preventing exposure of susceptible, healthy animals. Owners of herds of cattle in which the disease has not appeared should take every precaution to prevent its introduction. If it is necessary to introduce new animals into a herd, they should be procured from reputable breeders and it would be well to make special inquiry concerning Johne's disease. Such a breeder can usually furnish a statement from an accredited veterinarian concerning the health of the herd from which purchases are contemplated, with a specific statement in regard to clinical symptoms of Johne's disease. Though such precautions may seem un-necessary, it is much less expensive in both time and money to prevent the introduction of this insidious disease than to eradicate it after it becomes established in a herd.

The owner of any herd in which losses from Johne's disease are occurring should realize that, unless it is controlled, it is likely to become increasingly destructive until the herd becomes economically unprofitable. He should realize, too, that it is one of the most difficult of the infectious diseases to eradicate and that eradication will probably require at least 2 years of constant effort. The mere removal of cattle showing clinical symptoms will not usually bring relief, for too many apparently healthy animals are potential spreaders of the organisms. Although the johnin test is still not perfect, it has enough merit to justify its use in infected herds. The control programme that is most likely to succeed would include testing at regular intervals, preferably every 3 to 6 months; removing all reactors whether or not they were showing symptoms; cleaning and disinfecting thoroughly after any affected or reacting animal is removed from a barn or lot; and, most important of all, rearing young breeding stock in quarters that have not been used by mature animals.

Some cattle showing typical symptoms fail to react to the test. In any successful control programme all such animals must be considered sources of infection.

Stanchions, stalls, barns, pens and corrals in which affected cattle have been kept should be thoroughly cleaned and all wood or concrete mangers, drinking troughs and floors should be soaked for several hours in some disinfectant approved for tuberculosis-eradication work. Pens and corrals which have been used for such animals should have all the manure and at least 4 inches of the top-soil removed. This should be either buried or placed in a field to which cattle will not have access. Care should be taken that drainage from such a field does not contaminate pastures, streams or pens that may be used by healthy cattle.

Since the organisms of Johne's disease are excreted in the feces, special precautions should be taken to prevent contamination of any feed or water with cattle droppings. Cattle should not be allowed in feed alleys. Brooms for cleaning gutters, floors and stanchion platforms should be used for this purpose only and a different set should be used for the mangers, feed alleys and feed trucks. Care-takers should be careful not to contaminate hay, grain, silage or other feed with infective material carried on their feet. All too frequently herdsmen climb into a haymow or a silo without cleaning their boots or shoes.

Water from pools, ponds, sloughs and streams that receive surface drainage from lots or pastures that have been used by an infected herd is unsafe. On infected premises great care should be taken to prevent contamination of any pails or buckets from which young calves are to be fed.

During the past several years cattlemen have from time to time raised the question of the desirability of regulations requiring testing for Johne's disease as a prerequisite for interstate shipment. Livestock sanitary officials and authorities seem agreed that such a requirement is not now advisable because definite information that such tests are reliable is lacking. In several States indemnities for cattle slaughtered on account of Johne's disease are paid on the same basis as the indemnities for slaughtered tuberculous cattle. The Bureau of Animal Industry has been granted authority by Congress to pay indemnity to cattle, owners for animals that are slaughtered because of reaction to the Johnin test and the payments are made on the same basis as those on tuberculous cattle. Indemnity funds have been available for this purpose since July 1, 1927 and a number of livestock owners have received benefits from them.

Although specific figures are not available to prove it, many veterinarians and livestock sanitary officers believe that Johne's disease is increasing in the United States and that unless something is done to stop the increase the disease will become as serious a menace in this country as it is in some parts of Europe. Much more research is necessary, however, before definite knowledge that can be used to control and eradicate the disease completely will be available.

Chapter 3

BOVINE MASTITIS

W.T. Miller[1]

[1] *W.T. Miller is Veterinarian, Animal Disease Station, Bureau of Animal Industry.*

Bovine mastitis is responsible for enormous losses, through reduced milk production and in other ways, in our dairy herds. Here is a sound programme of control based on early detection of the disease, segregation of diseased cows and use of sanitary measures.

Bovine mastits is an extremely serious disease of dairy cattle. The annual economic loss to dairymen from loss of cows, decreased milk production and poor-quality milk is tremendous. In addition, certain human diseases can be contracted through the use of unpasteurized milk from affected cows. To reduce these losses and to improve both the quantity and quality of milk are of the greatest Importance at this time.

Mastitis moons inflammation of the udder from any cause. There are two forms of the disease, acute and chronic. The latter is the more common, but it is not readily recognized. The acute form, commonly known as garget, is familiar to every dairyman. The affected quarter is reddened, swollen, hot and painful. The secretion is very much reduced and varies from a watery, blood-tinged fluid containing a few solid particles to thick, yellow, ropy material.

In the past an attack of acute mastitis was thought to be temporary and it was believed that when it passed, recovery was complete. Actually, in most cases the acute symptoms represent a flare-up of the chronic form already present in the quarter. Recovery from an acute attack usually means a return to the chronic state.

When the average dairy herd is examined for mastitis, it is not unusual to find the chronic form of the disease in one or more quarters of the udders of half the cows. Because of the lack of easily recognized symptoms the owner may be unaware of the extent of the disease. On inquiry, however, the infected cows will be found to have had acute attacks, as a rule at the beginning or end of a lactation period. They are usually short milkers.

Mastitis is an infectious disease. Certain kinds of bacteria enter the opening into the teat canal, travel up the canal and lodge in the milk cistern at the base of the teat, where they cause a mild or low-grade inflammation. In the course of time the bacteria spread to other parts of the gland and the inflammation extends until finally the entire quarter is affected. Acute attacks usually occur as the infection progresses.

As a result of the inflammation, the composition of the milk is changed. Although the milk may appear normal, the percentages of butterfat, lactose (milk sugar), casein and possibly other elements are decreased. On the other hand the number of leucocytes, the salt content, the number of bacteria and the products resulting from inflammation and bacterial activity increase. A change in the character of the udder tissue itself also occurs. The normal secretory tissue is gradually replaced by nonsecretory, scar (fibrous) tissue. Finally the quarter loses its soft, pliable quality and hard areas, circumscribed or diffuse, appear in the vicinity of the milk cistern. In advanced cases the quarter becomes hardened throughout and there is an almost complete loss of secretory tissue.

With the change in the character of the udder tissue, milk production drops, which accounts for shortened lactation periods. The time required for this change to occur varies considerably, depending on the virulence of the invading bacteria, the natural resistance of the animal, the number of acute attacks and management and feeding practices. In some cases of chronic mastitis the animal may pass through a number of lactation periods before the disease manifests itself. On the other hand, many cows become entirely useless in a comparatively short time.

Bacteria Causing Mastitis

Bovine mastitis can be caused by a number of different kinds of bacteria. Of greatest importance are the streptococci, including several species that are responsible for such diseases in man as scarlet fever and septic sore throat. Fortunately, infection with these species occurs infrequently and usually as a result of the bacteria having been carried to the end of the teat on the hands of an infected milker. Bacteria of these species do not tend to spread through the herd. On the other hand the streptococci most commonly found in, mastitis rarely cause disease in man. However, they spread readily from cow to cow on the milker's hands or the cups of the milking machine. Once established these streptococci usually remain in the quarter for the rest of the life of the animal. An infected cow is therefore a constant source of danger for the other cows in the herd.

Next in importance as a cause of mastitis are the staphylococci. Several species are known and they undoubtedly cause many more cases of mastitis than is generally realized. Staphylococci, like streptococci, cause the chronic form of the disease, but they are not likely to persist in the udder for as long a time as the streptococci. Acute attacks which may terminate in the death of the animal occur frequently in staphylococcal mastitis.

Various other types of bacteria are found in occasional outbreaks of the disease. For the most part these types cause acute mastitis accompanied by systemic disturbance and not infrequently the animal dies. In most cases of this kind the infection leaves the udder after recovery. When these outbreaks occur, they constitute a serious problem through loss of function of quarters and death of cows. Fortunately they appear only sporadically.

Diagnosis

Early detection of diseased cows is extremely important. Acute attacks of mastitis can be diagnosed readily by clinical symptoms, but the chronic form presents some difficulty. Tests that largely solve this problem are now available. Diagnosis of mastitis in individual cows and recommendations for controlling the spread of the disease are functions of the veterinarian. Responsibility for carrying out sanitary measures, early detection of subsequent cases of. mastitis and proper disposition of diseased animals tests with the owner or herdsman. It is essential, therefore, that he should have some knowledge of the more common tests and understand their significance.

Tests for easy routine use must be easily applied and reasonably accurate. Two such tests are now in use in many herds. One is the strip-cup test. In this test several streams of milk are drawn from a quarter on to a fine-mesh wire screen immediately before the animal is milked. The appearance of clots or flakes or of watery or off-color milk on the screen is evidence of mastitis. As in other tests of similar nature, the accuracy of results obtained with the strip-cup test improves with frequent usage. To obtain best results the cup should be used before each milking or once a day at the very least. With this test mastitis can frequently be detected in previously healthy cows and bad milk Can be kept out of the general supply.

The second test is the bromthymol-blue or thybromol, test. Changes in the milk are detected by variations in color when the dye solution from which the test derives its name is mixed with it. Milk drawn from a healthy quarter is slightly acid. When a few drops of the dye are added to it, a pale yellowish-green color results. Milk from a diseased quarter is alkaline and this is indicated by a green color when the dye is added. Different shades of green may be encountered, depending on the degree of alkalinity. The more alkaline the milk, the darker the shade of green becomes. An intense yellow may be observed occasionally. This indicates a very acid condition and is usually accompanied by gross alteration in the appearance of the secretion. Frequent use of the brom-thymol-blue test also increases its effectiveness materially.

Prevention

Since curative measures are not entirely effective, a programme for controlling the spread of mbstitisaacteria from diseased to healthy cows affords an effective and practical means of dealing with the disease. In most cases the bacteria are carried on the milkers' hands or in the teat cups of the milking machine. When a healthy animal is milked immediately after an infected one, the mastitis bacteria are left on the teats of the healthy cow, in which repeated exposure will eventually produce the disease.

The purpose of the control programme, therefore, is to avoid exposure of healthy cows during milking. Detection of all cows with mastitis is the first step. Cows with extensive induration (hardening) of the udder should be removed immediately from the herd. They are unprofitable for milk production, are subject to recurrent acute attacks and provide a constant source of infection for other cows in the herd. The remaining diseased and healthy animals should then be separated into two groups. Complete segregation of the groups in separate barns with separate milkers is the most desirable arrangement. This is not absolutely necessary, however, if strict attention is given to the order of milking and other essential details of the programme.

The group of cows with healthy udders must always be milked before the infected group. When first-calf heifers are added to the herd, they should be placed with the clean cows unless they show signs of mastitis. Few heifers come into lactation infected with mastitis bacteria. Cows placed in the two groups should be maintained in them through subsequent lactation periods unless evidence of mastitis is found In members of the healthy group. Should the routine tests indicate the presence of mastitis in a healthy cow, it must be placed in the diseased group without delay. Once in the infected group, the animal must be kept there as long as it stays in the herd. Infected cows should be sold as soon as they become unprofitable or if they suffer recurrent acute attacks.

Certain sanitary measures must be included in the programme along with strict observance of the milking order. Individual cloths dipped in fresh hypochlorite solution (200 to 400 parts of chlorine per million) should be used to wipe the udder, teats and flanks of each cow before milking. These cloths must never be replaced in this solution after use. Between milkings they should be washed, sterilized by boiling or steaming and dried. After the cow is milked, each teat must be dipped in a small quantity of fresh hypochlorite solution of the strength indicated. This removes the drop of milk from the end of the teat and also repels flies. The solution should be discarded after being used for one cow.

Proper feeding must also be considered. Feeding a high-protein grain ration must be avoided, particularly for cows with mastitis or exposed to the disease. Such feed apparently overstimulates the udder and predisposes it to infection, while infected cows receiving such a ration are more subject to acute attacks and the secretion of abnormal milk. These recurrent attacks lead to more rapid deterioration of the udder. When cows with mild cases of chronic mastitis are fed and managed properly, they may remain in the herd for some time as profitable producers; but they must always be recognized as a source of danger to healthy cows.

Protection of the udder from injury and infection is of equal importance. Adequate stall space and ample bedding are absolute necessities to protect the teats and udder from being stepped on and from being bruised or chilled when the animals lie down. Floors and passageways should be so constructed as to give the cows good footing. To keep down infection, floors and stalls must be washed regularly and disinfected with 3- to 5-percent lye solution. As an additional safeguard, liberal use of lime or super-phosphate in back of the stalls and in the gutters is important.

Chapter 4

BLACKLEG

William M. Mohler[1]

[1] *William M. Mohler is Senior Veterinarian, Pathological Division, Bureau of Animal Industry.*

Blackleg, one of the most infectious of diseases and one that usually proves fatal, affects young cattle particularly. It can be prevented by vaccination. Proper disposal of animals that have died of the disease is very important.

Blackleg, also known as quarter ill, symptomatic anthrax, emphysematous anthrax and black quarter, is an acute infectious and usually fatal disease which attacks young cattle between 6 months and 2 years of age. Goats and sheeps are susceptible to and occasionally contract the disease, but other animals appear to be immune.

This disease is caused by *Clostridium chauvoei*, which is an anaerobic microorganism, that is, one that develops rapidly only in the absence of oxygen. These organisms are in the form of short rods and produce spores that are very resistant to destruction by heat, cold, drying or chemical disinfectants. Usually the organism gains entrance into the body of the animal through small cuts or punctures in the skin; large cuts or open wounds are not favorable for growth of the organism. In some cases the organism may enter the body through abrasions in the mucous membranes of the tongue, mouth cavity or throat.

In localities where blackleg occurs frequently, it is the young cattle, especially those between the ages of 6 and 18 months, that are usually infected. Calves 4 to 5 months old sometimes become infected, but an increase in the number of cases is noted with an increase in age. Very young animals evidently have an inherited or natural immunity which gradually wears off as they approach 6 months of age. The disease is seldom contracted by cattle past 2 years of age and almost absolute immunity is noted after 3 years.

Symptoms

The symptoms of blackleg are so characteristic that it is possible to recognize the disease easily. The first symptoms to be noted are high fever, loss of appetite and a suspension of rumination, followed by great depression. Breathing becomes more rapid than normal. In most cases the animal has difficulty in moving about and it frequently lies down. Rapidly developing swellings or tumors in the tissues under the skin are characteristic. They may appear on the neck and shoulders, beneath the breast and on the flanks and thighs and in some instances they appear on the gums, the base of the tongue and the wall of the pharynx. The tumors are accompanied by severe febrile symptoms. At first small and painful to the touch, they rapidly increase in size and may cover a considerable part of the body. Upon pressure the tumors make a peculiar crackling sound which is due to the collection of gas formed by the causative micro-organisms.

As the swellings increase in size, the symptoms become more intense. The temperature may reach 107° F and the respiration may increase to 140 or more a minute. The animal is unable to rise, the extremities become cold and the temperature usually falls and may become sub-normal shortly before death. Violent convulsions and trembling of the muscles are noted before death. Although there are some recoveries, death generally occurs in 12 to 36 hours after the first appearance of the disease.

The carcass of an animal dead from blackleg soon becomes distended by gas, partly through fermentation in the gastrointestinal. tract and partly through the formation of gas in the tissue under the skin. Marked distention is noted in the region of the blackleg tumors and where there is loose tissue, especially between the shoulder and the chest and on the outer surface of the hindquarters. In many instances this distention causes the legs on the upper side to stand out straight from the body. Shortly after death a dark, blood-colored, frothy discharge flows from the nostrils and anus. An incision made through the skin into the affected muscle tissue fails to demonstrate any decomposition, but it is possible to detect a characteristic sweetishsour odor.

The skin covering the blackleg tumors is affected with dry gangrene. The distended muscle, which are easily torn, are dark brown or black and the spaces surrounding them are filled with bloody liquid and gas. The blood in the badly affected parts of the body is thick and charged with gas and has a disagreeable odor. In the remaining parts of the carcass the blood is normal and coagulates easily after death, forming a solid clot. Hemorrhages are found on the heart and lungs. The spleen is always normal, but congestion is noted in the liver.

Thus it may be seen that a post-mortem examination should serve to distinguish blackleg from other diseases. Nevertheless, though a diagnosis may be made at autopsy, it is sometimes-advisable to send specimens from affected animals to the laboratory for a conclusive diagnosis.

Treatment and Prevention

Medicinal treatment of animals has thus far proved unavailing. The only reliable and effective means known for protecting animals against blackleg is vaccination, which has been thoroughly tried and proved to be reliable.

Vaccines for protection against blackleg have been greatly improved in recent years. Those produced at the present time include blackleg bacterin, natural aggressin, cultural aggressin, cultural vaccine and tissue vaccine. These vaccines are used extensively in the United States and give excellent results, as they confer immunity without producing any vaccination disease.

As vaccine is a preventive and not a curative agent, it is useless to vaccinate an animal after the symptoms of blackleg have developed. The immunity conferred by vaccination varies according to the kind of vaccine used and may last 12 to 18 months or longer.

Antiblackleg serum is produced for treating calves already affected with blackleg, as well as for creating a temporary passive immunity in exposed animals in an infected herd. At present the product is rarely used in the United States, but if it is available at the onset of the disease it may be efficacious in some cases.

When blackleg occurs on a ranch or farm it is of the utmost importance that owners of cattle in the district realize that every animal affected with the disease may be the means of propagating and disseminating the infection. Losses may not occur immediately on infected premises; in some cases they occur only after a lapse of years. It is recommended, therefore, that every effort be made to reduce the danger of infection by taking appropriate measures to dispose of all dead animals and with them the infection they carry. The carcass should be entirely destroyed by burning if this is possible. Otherwise a hole 6 feet deep should be dug and the body placed therein and well covered with quicklime before the earth is filled in. Any place where the animal was lying should be thoroughly sprinkled with a strong disinfectant, such as a solution of commercial lye and hydrated lime (2½ pounds of lye and 2½ pounds of lime in 8½ gallons of water).

The eradication of blackleg infection from pastures is difficult. In most cases it is impossible to pasture livestock on other land long enough for the infection to die out. It appears, therefore, that vaccination is the only practicable and effective means of protecting cattle against blackleg. If vaccine is used year alter year to prevent the development of new cases over a long period, it is possible that the old infection will finally disappear.

Chapter 5

SHIPPING FEVER OR HEMORRHAGIC SEPTICEMIA

C.D. Stein[1]

[1] *C.D. Stein is Associate Veterinarian, Pathological Division, Bureau of Animal Industry.*

The author calls this the most serious of a group of cattle maladies that are commonly associated with the hardships and hazards of shipping–that is, the handling, neglect or exposure of animals in transit or shortly afterward. It is an infectious disease which often terminates in death. The losses from shipping fever can be greatly reduced by careful management in shipping. Vaccination with bacterins at least 10 days before shipping or injection of antiserum may reduce losses.

Shipping fever or stockyard fever, is an infectious disease of cattle usually attended with a high mortality. Its medical name, "hemorrhagic septicemia," was given it because it is a septicemia or poisoning, of the blood (and hence often runs a short, fatal course) and hemorrhages in the body tissues and organs of animals dead from the disease are usually an outstanding characteristic.

The disease occurs in cattle in all parts of the United States. The losses appear to be greatest among young animals, especially those, that are thin and poorly nourished. A large number of outbreaks of hemorrhagic septicemia in cattle are associated with the shipment of animals from one point to another by rail or truck and their passage through public stockyards. The vitality of an animal is lowered by the hardships of transit and its resistance to infection is decreased. The disease is therefore a serious problem to both shippers and receivers of cattle. In some years very considerable losses occur, whereas in other years they maybe slight.

It is generally believed that weather conditions influence the prevalence of the disease, since cattle appear to suffer from it most in the fall, winter and early spring during particularly changeable or inclement weather. After prolonged travel under such weather conditions, for example, they may arrive on the farm of the purchaser in a run-down condition, though they had appeared perfectly healthy when purchased in the stockyards. Overcrowding, irregularity in feeding and watering, hard driving, lack of rest and proper shelter and the general excitement associated with shipping are other devitalizing factors that may play a part in reducing normal vigor and increasing the susceptibility to shipping fever.

Cause

The primary cause of hemorrhagic septicemia in cattle has not been definitely determined and there is a difference of opinion both among practicing veterinarians and among research workers.

According to the older school of thought, the principal causative factor is the germ *Pasteurella baviseptica.* The organism has been found in the air passages of normal animals and organisms closely resembling it are widely distributed in nature. The theory is that such organisms become virulent under certain conditions and that animals harboring them readily develop so-called shipping fever when their natural resistance is lowered.

According to the newer school of thought, the hemorrhagic septicemia organism probably plays a secondary role, like that of diphtheroids, streptoocci and *Bacillus coli* organisms and there is another primary infective agent concerned in the production of the disease. The nature of this agent is not known, but it is thought by some to be a virus. When cattle are received after a hard rail road journey many of them may manifest symptoms of the disease and local stock that come in contact with the affected animals very often become infected. Just what part the contamination of yards, buildings and equipment by affected cattle plays in setting up the disease in non-infected animals is not known, but undoubtedly this is a source of danger. It is worthy of note that the co-existence of two factors (a virus and a bacterium) as necessary causative agents in certain infectious diseases has been recognized in recent years, notably in the case of swine influenza.

Symptoms and Lesions

Shipping fever in cattle usually develops very rapidly and lasts from 2 to 8 days or longer. Affected animals first show an elevation of body temperature, ranging from 104° to 107° F, accompanied by loss of appetite, mucopurulent discharge from the nose, an occasional hacking cough, swollen, watery eyes, general depression, gaunt appearance, stiffened gait and sometimes diarrhoea (Fig. 1). Within 3 to 5 days after the first symptoms appear, affected animals may develop pneumonia and die in 48 to 72 hours; or the disease may assume a chronic course and the sick animals may linger on for several weeks. In mild attacks, affected animals may recover if a week or two.

During the course of the disease other symptoms may occur. Swelling may appear beneath the skin of the head, throat or dewlap.

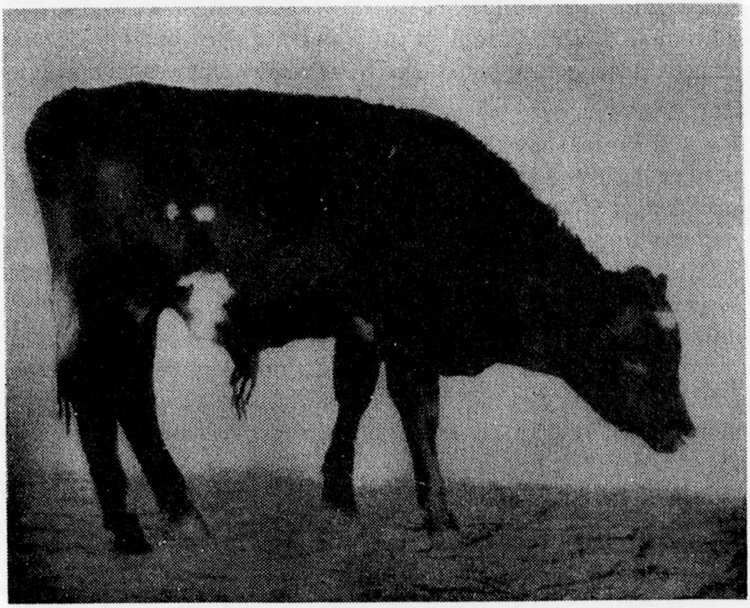

Fig. 1: A steer affected with hemorrhagic septicemia, showing typical attitude of dejection.

These enlargements are somewhat soft and pit on pressure. The tongue is often extensively swollen and the animal drools and slobbers because of the irritation to its tongue and throat. There may be difficulty in breathing, depending on the degree of involvement of the air passages and the lungs. Muscular trembling may be evident. There may be a blood-stained discharge from the nostrils and strings of mucus may hang from the mouth. Examination of the nostrils often reveals the presence of many small hemorrhages or blood spots, just beneath their lining membranes.

There is an intestinal form of the disease in which the changes are found chiefly in the abdominal cavity. This form may develop after the disease has appeared in the lungs. The stomach, intestines and kidneys and the lymph glands belonging to them become studded with hemorrhages of various sizes and the intestines become Intensely inflamed. Diarrhoea sets in and shreds of mucus and bloody droppings are passed. The intestinal form is rare; most cases show severe involvement of the lungs and the symptoms of croupous pneumonia. The animals may stand with their forelegs wide apart in order to breathe more freely. They lose flesh very rapidly, their abdomens become "tucked up," and the eyes quickly become sunken. A staggering gait, caused by extreme weakness, is sometimes noticed.

On postmortem examination the following anatomical changes may be observed in the carcass of an animal dead of hemorrhagic septicemia: Swellings of doughy consistency, containing jellylike material tinged with blood, may be found under the skin. If these swellings occur in the region of the shoulder or flank, they are sometimes mistaken for those of blackleg. The lymph glands are enlarged and hemorrhagic (injected with blood). The mucous membranes lining the nose, throat and air passages of the lungs are inflamed and may contain blood-stained mucus. Hemorrhages may be observed in the fat tissue around the kidneys and in the serous membranes of the internal organs.

When the disease is chiefly in the chest, the lungs are darkened in color and their fibrous tissues are much thickened owing to the collection of bloody serum in their meshes. There may be solidification of one or more lobes (pneumonia). The diaphragm, heart sac and heart walls show numerous bloody points and larger collections of blood.

In the intestinal form, hemorrhages of the intestines are present and there is sloughing of the lining of the intestinal wall, as a result of which the intestinal contents are wrapped in a covering of bloody mucus.

In acute forms of the disease the animals may die suddenly and in such cases the changes are not very marked although bacteriological examination of the body fluids may demonstrate the presence of hemorrhagic septicemia organisms.

Diagnosis

It is often difficult to diagnose hemorrhagic septicemia because of its similarity to certain other disease conditions encountered in cattle. Owing to its acute course, high fever and rapid termination, the disease may be mistaken for anthrax, malignant edema or blackleg. While certain characteristic features of these diseases may aid in making a tentative diagnosis, a bacteriologic examination which includes both cultural tests and inoculation of laboratory animals is sometimes necessary to detect the nature of the disease and especially to differentiate it from others.

Other conditions in cattle, such as coccidiosis, cornstalk disease, lead poisoning, sweetclover poisoning and other forms of vegetable poisoning, may be mistaken for hemorrhagic septicemia. In an outbreak of suspected hemorrhagic septicemia, diagnosis, treatment and methods of control should be left to an experienced veterinarian.

Control and Prevention

In considering measures for the control and prevention of this disease, it is important to remember that hemorrhagic septicemia is the most serious of a group of cattle maladies that commonly result from mishandling, neglect or exposure of animals in transit or shortly after their arrival at their destination. Hence the elimination of predisposing factors, such as overdriving, overcrowding, overfeeding and lack of rest, water, feed and proper shelter during transit, is stressed. Suggestions for reduction of losses due to hemorrhagic septicemia and other diseases of cattle incident to shipping will be found in the following recommendations from United States, Department of Agriculture Leaflet 38, Maintaining the Health of Livestock in Transit.[2]

---

[2] MILLER, A.W. MAINTAINING THE HEALTH OF LIVESTOCK IN TRANSIT, U.S. Dept. Agr. Leaflet 88, 8 pp, illus. 1931 (Revised).

Avoid hard driving and allow ample time for rest before loading. On arrival at the pens, the animals should not be allowed to fill up on water, but should first have rest and be fed some native grass or non legume hay.

Avoid overcrowding cattle in the cars. In cold weather, bed the car well. In very severe weather, in northern latitudes, it may be well to line the side walls of the car with heavy paper, especially if the cattle are young or unthrifty.

Give feed and water at proper intervals en route. When unloaded for feed, water and rest, the cattle should have plenty of time to become well rested.

Under the 28-hours law 5 hours' rest is the minimum specified time and the railroads ordinarily allow that period, exclusive of the time of unloading and reloading. It is better, however, to give stocker and feeder cattle special care, allowing at least 8 hours for feed, water and rest. * * * Cows in an advanced stage of pregnancy, commonly termed "springers," should receive particular attention.

The common practice of withholding water from animals until they are very thirsty so that later they will take a heavy fill is harmful. It tends to upset the digestive system so seriously that the animals are slow in resuming normal feeding and gain in weight. It is therefore recommended that this damaging practice be discontinued through general agreement among livestock owners and handlers.

In the case of stocker and feeder cattle that pass through the public market, the same attention should be given to the shipments back to the country that has been outlined for the shipments to market. Following the arrival of cattle at their final destination in the country, they should receive special attention and care to help them over the period of lowered vitality resulting from the hardships of travel.

Feeder cattle on arrival should be given a fill of dry roughage, such as timothy hay, prairie hay or corn stover. After having access to this roughage a few hours, they should have water, but not all they will drink. By the end of the first day, give free access to dry roughage and water.

Most feeder cattle are raised on grasses different from those found in the fattening areas. Therefore, if they are to be pasture fed, let them become accustomed to the new grasses gradually, giving them at first only a few hours' grazing each day, especially if the grass is still green.

If feeder cattle are intended for dry-lot feeding with no pasture available, give them access to cornstalk fields or feed them on corn fodder and hay for from 10 days to 2 weeks before starting them on the fattening rations.

If the cattle arrive in cold weather, especially if it is wet and stormy, provide adequate dry shelter. Severe exposure to cold and dampness combined, during the period of low vitality, is liable to have very serious results. If there is any sign of sickness, segregate diseased animals and keep them quiet.

The use of biological products to prevent hemorrhagic septicemia or to control outbreaks has been successful in many instances, but unsatisfactory results have followed in some outbreaks.

The biological products used are either preventive (bacterin and aggressin) or curative (antiserum). Bacterins or aggressins increase the animal's resistance against hemorrhagic septicemia infection, They produce an active immunity of long duration, usually several, months to a year. It is believed that a high degree of immunity is established in 10 days to 2 weeks after vaccination with either bacterin or aggressin.

For best results feeder and stocker cattle should be treated with bacterin or aggressin at least 10 days before shipment, as the use of these products on animals in transit or a few days after they reach their destination appears to be of little or no value, according to experimental work by the Bureau of Animal Industry and other agencies.[3]

---

[3] To ascertain the value of vaccination in reducing losses from hemorrhagic septicemia in animals in transit, the Bureau of Animal Industry, in cooperation with traders and livestock exchanges, conducted experimental work in the control of hemorrhagic septicemia at certain stockyards in 1924 and 1925. During 1924, 151, 475 feeder and stocker cattle were vaccinated by veterinary inspectors. During 1925, in an experiment in which 4,439 animals were handled, 2,234 were vaccinated with aggressin and 2,205 were shipped to their destination without treatment, as controls. The results of these experiments based on incomplete reports received from owners of treated and untreated cattle indicate that the administration of bacterin or aggressin confers little if any immunity on animals in transit, many of which apparently have the disease in the incubative stage. In fact, some of the evidence tends to show that losses were greater in the animals treated with aggressin than in those untreated.

On the other hand, the administration of antihemorrhagic septicemia immune serum, which contains great numbers of immune bodies, produces an immediate increase in resistance to the disease. This is, however, a passive immunity of short duration, lasting only a few weeks.

Since antihemorrhagic septicemia serum furnishes quick protection and also has some curative value, its use in preference to bacterin or aggressin is indicated for treatment of cattle in transit or within a few days after they arrive at their destination, particularly if some of the animals in the shipment show symptoms of the disease.

Anaphyloxis (shock or severe reactions) may sometimes follow the administration of antiserum or bacterins. To avoid this, only homologous serum (that is, serum obtained from bovine species) should be used and bacterins should preferably be composed of a bacterial suspension in normal (0.8 percent) saline solution free from toxic broth or other foreign protein.

The advisability of using biological products and their administration should be left to a competent veterinarian.

Tests conducted by the Bureau of Animal Industry have shown that both laboratory animals and cattle can be immunized under experimental conditions against hemorrhagic septicemia by either aggressin or bacterin. Cattle, sheep and laboratory animals can also be immunized by treatment with weakened (attenuated) cultures.

During these experiments, animals vaccinated with aggressin and subsequently exposed to artificial infection remained well. Animals treated with aggressin developed immunity to artificial exposure in as short a period as 4 days, while those treated with bacterin required 9 days to develop immunity. Cattle were found to be resistant to infection 15 months after vaccination with aggressin.

In most cases medicinal treatment of a fully established case of shipping fever is of little value. In visibly sick animals, especially during the early stages of the disease, the administration of large doses of antihemorrhagic septicemia serum (one or two injections of 50 cubic centimeters or more) frequently assists in bringing about recovery. All apparently well animals should be removed from sick ones and placed in separate, noninfected quarters. If new cases develop among them a few days after their removal, the remaining healthy ones should be removed again to another locality. In that way the unaffected animals can be kept out of danger of further contamination.

The administration of sodium bicarbonate has been reported by some stockmen and veterinarians as being of considerable value in both the treatment and the prevention of this disease, During 1934, 1935 and 1936, sodium bicarbonate administered in the form of a drench, on the feed or in drinking water at the rate of 1 ounce to each 100 pounds of body weight, was given once a day for 14 days by stockmen and stockyard officials to several thousand cattle. Some of the animals were treated in the stockyards and others after arrival on the home premises following shipment. A large number of untreated animals in both groups were held as controls. Reports received by the Bureau on the results of this treatment showed little difference between the treated and untreated animals in their resistance to shipping fever.

Since hemorrhagic septicemia is an infectious disease, the carcasses of animals that have died of it should be burned or buried. Premises are usually contaminated by infected cattle that have recently passed through some of the larger markets. All stables sheds or yards that have contained infected animals should be disinfected. The interior of the stables, especially the mangers and gutters, should be washed with a disinfectant, such as compound cresol solution, 4 ounces to a gallon of water or carbolic acid, 6 ounces to a gallon of water. For dairy barns, however, where the odor of these disinfectants would be objectionable, milk of lime or some other nonodorous disinfectant may be preferred. The yards may be disinfected by the application of a solution made of 5 ounces of copper sulfate to a gallon of water. The best way to apply disinfectant solutions is with a spray pump such as is used in spraying orchard trees. All refuse and waste material from the stable and barnyard should be removed to a place not accessible to cattle or sheep the manure should be spread on fields and plowed under. A plentiful supply of light and air should be provided for the contaminated stables. Open fields or pastures are cleansed rapidly by the action of sunlight.

Chpater 6

MILK FEVER

L.T. Giltner[1]

[1] *L.T. Giltner is Senior Veterinarian, Pathological Division, Bureau of Animal Industry.*

Milk fever, which causes the collapse and sudden death of high-producing dairy cows at the time of calving, is always accompanied by a serious unbalance in the mineral content of the blood. Treatment by a veterinarian, as described in this article, is an almost certain cure.

Milk fever, also called parturient paresis and parturient hypocalcemia, is an affection of cows occurring shortly after calving. It is characterized by paralysis of the motor and sensory nervous apparatus. Despite its name, milk fever usually is not accompanied by fever. There is always, however, a marked and rapid lowering of the blood calcium, so that the name "parturient hypocalcemia," which means too little calcium at calving time, is quite appropriate.

Milk fever is one of the most common, widespread and serious of the acute of afflictions of dairy cows. It affects almost exclusively the high-producing better nourished animals. It very rarely occurs at the first calving; sometimes at the second calving; and most frequently after the birth of the third to seventh calf or during the prime of life. The poorly nourished cow is seldom a victim and difficult calving (dystocia) is hardly ever followed by milk fever. After the first attack, the trouble may recur at one or more subsequent calvings.

Cause

The early investigations into the cause and nature of milk fever are of considerable interest to the present-day student for the light they throw on developments in medical science. Most veterinary writers today begin their discussions of the earlier studies of the disease with the work done late in the nineteenth and in the early part of the present century, when the theory of bacterial infection and systemic intoxication with bacterial toxins associated in some manner with parturition was in vogue. In 1897, Schmidt, a Danish veterinarian, acting on the theory that milk fever resulted from infection of the udder, experimented with injections of a solution of potassium iodide into the udders of cows sick with the disease. Although this treatment proved remarkably successful in his hands, it did not afford a satisfactory explanation of his infection theory, since he later found that when air was introduced into the udder along with the potassium iodide solution equally good results were obtained. In the early years of the present century it was found that oxygen or filtered air alone proved superior to the potassium iodide solution as a treatment. Bacteriologic investigations soon showed conclusively that milk fever was decidedly not a bacterial infection of the udder. However, Schmidt's treatment or a modification of it–the injection of filtered air into the udder–proved so effective that no further investigations into the cause of the disease were undertaken at that time, since researches on other diseases were deemed more important.

All excellent treatment had been discovered and when it was carried out skillfully, especially with strict aseptic precautions, milk fever could be readily controlled or at least when cases occurred they could be cured. Research workers were apparently content to let matters stand, even though the underlying cause of the strange malady remained obscure.

Finally, however, in 1925, Dryerre and Greig[2] proposed the theory that milk fever is an expression of an acute deficiency of calcium in the blood. Studies of the blood of cows affected with the disease revealed that there was a marked fall from the normal calcium

---

[2] DRYERRE, HENRY, and GREIG, J. RUSSELL. MILK FEVER: ITS POSSIBLE ASSOCIATION WITH DERANGEMENTS IN THE INTERNAL SECRETIONS. Vet. Rec. 5: [225]-231, 1925.

level. Moreover, when calcium in the form of calcium gluconate solution was infected intravenously in an appropriate dose into cows suffering from milk fever, a cure was promptly effected. Why then, does inflation of the udder with potassium iodide, oxygen or filtered air have a curative effect? Greig[3] explains this as follows: "The effect is a mechanical one in that it elicits mammary distention and so prevents the further interchange of calcium from the blood to the gland acini (the microscopic saclike elements of the gland). There is also reason to believe that the calcium, which is heavily concentrated in the gland, is forced back into the blood as the result of the mammary distention."

Chemical studies have revealed other abnormalities in the blood of rattle suffering from milk fever. In some cases hypermagnesemia (increase in blood magnesium) has been found, in others, hypomagnesemia (decrease in blood magnesium). A decrease in phosphorus and an increase in blood sugar (hyperglycemia) have also been observed.

In the normal animal all of the various blood constituents are maintained at a very constant level through the proper coordination of the body's complex and delicate glandular mechanism. The discovery of the changes in the blood brought about by the disordered functioning of this mechanism during milk fevelr has been of immense importance in pointing the way to effective treatment, but the basic causes of the break-down of the mechanism have not yet been fully brought to light.

Symptoms

The earliest stages in the development of an attack of milk fever are frequently not noted or pass unrecognized by the casual observer. The first symptoms, depression and disinclination to move about or to eat, may set in as early as 6 hours after calving, but more often they begin anytime from about the twelfth hour to the third or fourth day. Although milk fever symptoms may at times appear before parturition or even several weeks afterwards, such causes may be involved with other, affections common to the parturient or post-parturient state and the diagnosis should be confirmed by laboratory

---

3 GREIG, J. RUSSELL. THE NATURE OF MILK FEVEB. 11th Internatl. Vet. Cong. Rpt. 3: 306-324, illus. 1930.

aid. Cases have been observed in which the animal appeared excited and highly nervous for a short time, with twitching of the muscles and jerking of the legs and head, but the classical picture of milk fever begins, as already stated, with depression and this is followed by collapse and complete loss of consciousness. The animal lies with its head turned to one side, the eyes are dull and expressionless, the membrane covering the eye is reddened, the muzzle is dry, the extremities are cold and the body temperature is usually below normal.

Udall[4] states that one of the most constant and characteristic signs in milk fever is a tonic spasm of the muscles of the neck, giving the neck a distinct lateral kink. This symptom is seen more frequently then the turning of the head to the side. Throughout an attack the animal ceases to feed or ruminate and an body functions are at low ebb. The pulse and breathing are accelerated, the breathing often being labored and accompanied by groaning. Bloating is not uncommon. The most frequent complications of milk fever are pneumonia, which generally occurs as a result of inhaling food material regurgitated from the paunch while the animal is lying down and septic inflammation of the womb from various causes. Animals that are not appropriately treated usually die within several hours to a few days.

Prevention and Treatment

Among the serious cattle plagues, milk fever is unique in that its treatment when properly carried out is remarkably successful, while practical and effective preventive measures are lacking. Of the suggested means of prevention, the injection of a solution of a calcium salt directly after calving is worthy of mention, as is also the practice of partial instead of complete milking during the first several days after calving. Obviously, however, the former procedure is more or less experimental and not practical and the latter may lead to mastitis. Special measures should be taken to insure an adequate ration for and proper care of the pregnant and parturient cow.

As already mentioned, however, there are two methods of treatment that are efficacious if properly carried out, but to insure

---

[4] UDALL, D.H. THE PRACTICE OF VETERINARY MEDICINE. Ed. 3, 672 pp. illus. Ithaca, N.Y. 1939.

success, treatment must be instituted as early as possible. The procedure preferred by veterinarians consists in intravenously injecting calcium gluconate in 20 per cent solution. It is sometimes necessary to repeat the injection one or more times to effect a cure. Solutions of other calcium salts may also be used, but care must be taken that the solution does not enter the tissues surrounding the vein, since this causes severe irritation, often leading to swellings or sloughing. The injection should not be made under the skin.

The alternate procedure, consisting of inflation of the udder with filtered air, must be undertaken with great care so as to avoid introducing infection by contaminating the teat canal. Equipment must be kept sterile and ready for use at all times. Before beginning the actual inflation, a clean sterile cloth is placed under the udder, the udder and the teats are cleansed with warm soapy water and dried with a sterile towel and the teats and their orifices are disinfected. Each quarter is fully distended with air and the teat is tied with a flat tape or bandage which is removed after not more than 3 or 4 hours. During an attack the animal should not be permitted to lie on its side, since there is danger of pneumonia from inhaling regurgitated paunch contents; bracing the animal so that it rests on its brisket will prevent this.

Usually with either the calcium-injection or the air-inflation treatment the response is rapid. In complicated cases the animal returns to consciousness in less than an hour and is often on its feet in 2 to 4 hours after treatment. The body temperature and the digestive and eliminatory functions return to normal, as evidenced by the resumption of rumination, defecation and urination. In certain cases both procedures may be used, the one assisting the other in bringing about recovery. When medication in addition to the calcium salts is deemed necessary, the veterinarian always administers it by the vein or hypodermically and not by a drench, since there is danger that the medic me might pass down the windpipe and cause pneumonia. When treatments fail it is usually because there are complications, such as septic inflammation of the womb, pneumonia or some serious involvement of the digestive organs.

Chapter 7

MISCELLANEOUS DISEASES OF CATTLE

G.T. Creech, R.L. Knudson & O.L. Osteen[1]

[1] *G.T. Creech is Senior Veterinarian, R.L. Knudson is Assistant Veterinarian and O.L. Osteen is Associate Veterinarian, Pathological Division, Bureau of Animal Industry. The sections on White Scours, Acetonemia and Pseudorabies were prepared by Dr. Knudson and those on Calf Diphtheria, Pneumonia and Choke by Dr. Osteen.*

Here is information regarding the nature, causes, symptoms, prevention and control of white scours, acetonemia, pseudorabies (mad itch), common warts, epithelioma (cancer eye), tumors of the lymph glands (lymphocytoma), lumpy jaw (actinomycosis and actinobacillosis), nasal granuloma (snoring disease) and specific ophthalmia (pinkeye).

White Scours (Infectious Diarrhoea or Acute Dysentery)

The condition Commonly referred to as white scours is an acute, contagious, infectious disease of young or newborn calves, characterized by a profuse diarrhoea an rapid exhaustion. The majority of animals affected are very young, less than 5 days old; the disease is not uncommon in calves less than 48 hours old. In severe outbreaks, however, it has been known to spread to older calves. The percentage of recoveries is very small, with or without treatment.

White scours is primarily an infectious diarrhoea that later affects the entire system. The disease is due to an invasion of the intestinal tract by certain types of microorganisms, particularly varieties of the colon bacillus, which are widely distributed in nature.

Outbreaks of this disease may occur at any season of the year, but it is most common in stabled animals during the fall and winter months. In some cases it may begin in the fall and increase in severity and in number of animals affected until spring.

Infection may take place through either the navel cord or the digestive tract. Calves may become infected in various ways during birth, by sucking a contaminated udder, from the contaminated hands of attendants, by exposure to contaminated stable litter or by contact with sick calves in nearby pens. These possible sources of infection should be kept in mind in relation to control measures to be discussed later.

Symptoms of the disease vary somewhat in individual cases. At birth, the calf may appear normal or occasionally it may be weak or dull, but in 48 to 72 hours or later, a profuse yellowish-white diarrhoea with a very pungent and disagreeable odor develops. At the same time it may be noticed that the animal appears dull and listless. The eyes may be drawn back in the sockets and lack luster. Stiffness of gait is not uncommon. The hair coat quite often appears rough and the skin dry. The hindquarters may be covered with the discharge from the bowels and in severe cases there may be loss of hair over the parts affected, with considerable irritation and inflammation of the skin. The abdomen may show a tucked-up or gaunt appearance in very young calves, while in older animals there may be more or less distention from large quantities of milk previously consumed. Affected calves have a tendency to sleep much of the time and the appetite is very poor. Depending upon the severity of the attack, there may be increasing prostration until death ensues, While all or a part of the symptoms described are seen in the majority of cases, in some instances there may be a rather sudden attack, the animal dying in a few hours and occasionally a calf may be found dead without any definite signs of previous illness.

In making a diagnosis of this disease, it is at times quite difficult to distinguish between white scours and diarrhoea due to other causes, particularly those of a dietary nature, such as overfeeding, irregular feeding, use of unclean utensils, feeding cold milk and too rapid changes in feed or exposure to cold drafts and cold damp floors. When a number of calves are affected, as a precautionary measure the contagious form of white scours should always be considered as a possibility until diagnosed as some other form of diarrhoea.

A calf that has succumbed to white scours win show soiled hindquarters from the bowel discharges and the carcass will be emaciated. An odor peculiar to the disease may also be noticed. On autopsy, small hemorrhages may be found on the serous linings-thin lining membranes–of the body cavities and also in the region of the heart. There seems to be a localization of lesions or tissue changes, in the digestive tract and slight to severe hemorrhages will be found on the lining of the stomach and small intestine. There may be varying amounts of free blood in the bowel. The contents of the intestinal tract are a dirty yellowish-gray color and have a fetid odor. The intestines may be distended with gas. Varying amounts of a red-colored fluid may be present in the body cavities. It is probable that not all the tissue changes described will be present in each individual case, those occurring depending somewhat on the severity of the infection and the length of time the animal has been affected. In some instances marked lesions may be absent, whereas in long continued cases there may be infection of the joints, pneumonia and inflammation of the serous linings of the body cavities. Foreign substances, such as bedding and hair, may be found in the stomach.

Prevention and Control Measures

Medicinal treatment begun after the onset of diarrhoeal symptoms is usually of little avail. A hyperimmune calf-scour serum given as a preventive treatment soon after birth will aid in preventing heavy losses but is of little value after infection has taken place. In some instances a bacterin (made of killed organisms) has been used to inoculate pregnant cows, but little is known regarding the efficacy of such treatment at the present time.

In combating this disease, the owner should remember that the all important thing is to prevent primary, infection of the newborn calf. This can be accomplished only by strict sanitary measures that is, by providing the greatest possible cleanliness at the time of birth and during the first few days of life, when the animal is most susceptible to the infection. A large box stall or maternity stall that can be readily cleaned and disinfected at frequent intervals should be provided for the cow at the time of parturition. Shortly before the time of calving, the external genitals, hindquarters, tail and udder should be thoroughly cleaned and disinfected with a 3 percent solution of liquor cresolis compositus. Just before the udder is disinfected, a few streams of milk should be drawn into a vessel (not onto the stable floor) and discarded. As soon as possible after the calf is delivered, its navel should be disinfected with fresh tincture of iodine. Also, before the calf suckles, its mouth may be washed out with a 4 percent solution of boric acid.

The maternity stall should be kept clean by periodic removal of an litter and frequent renewal of the bedding. This is very important, as most calves have a habit of chewing the bedding or other foreign substances and the infective organisms may this gain entrance to the digestive tract. It is well known that the first instinct of a normal calf is to obtain food from its mother. This first food is colostral milk, the secretion of the mammary gland of the cow immediately after calving. Colostrum is somewhat different in composition from milk that is secreted later; it aids in cleaning out the digestive tract and also gives the calf resistance against harmful bacteria that may gain entrance to the intestinal canal.

The adoption of some system of regular feeding of calves is essential, since even in an apparently healthy calf an overloaded stomach may result in severe indigestion, which may lower its resistance to such an extent that it becomes susceptible to the causative agent of white scours. Once the infection has gained a foothold in the herd, it is likely to spread to other calves in the same group.

A plan for the care and feeding of very young calves is as follows: For the first 12 hours the calf remains with the dam and obtains colostrum without restraint, since, as a general rule, the calf is not strong enough to overeat. At the end of 12 hours a muzzle is applied and all feed withheld for 24 hours. For 30 days the muzzle is not removed except while the calf is feeding. The allowance of the dam's milk for the first feeding day is 5 to 6 percent of the calf's body weight. This is divided into three feedings, to each of which is added an equal amount of limewater. The mixture is heated to 100° F. and fed in a sterilized pail. For the second feeding day, the quantity of dam's milk to be given is 6 or 7 percent of the calf's weight.

The amount of limewater at each feeding should never be more than 1 pint. At the end of the first week, the calf may receive a quantity of milk daily equal to 8 to 12 percent of its body weight. Feed is given in individual pails morning, noon and night, with a pint of limewater at each feeding. The pails should always be cleaned and sterilized before being used.

It may be advisable during the first week to take the calf's temperature every day before the noon feeding. If it is 103° F. or more, give an enema, using a 1 percent solution of liquor cresolis compositus and administer 3 ounces of liquid petrolatum by mouth. Feed should be withheld until the temperature is normal.

Calves showing symptoms of the disease should be isolated; their feces, which contain the infective agent, should be destroyed; and the stables should be frequently disinfected. Also, all tools and equipment used around the pens should be cleaned and disinfected. The sick calves should be given a dose of 4 to 6 ounces of castor oil, followed by 1 ounce of sodium bicarbonate in a half pint of water, combined with 3 drams of aromatic spirits of ammonia. Coffee may be given as a stimulant and the strength of the calf can be preserved by feeding raw eggs in pasteurized milk. Limewater may be given at frequent intervals. Decoctions of linseed, barley, oats, etc., may also be given. From 5 to 10 drops of liquor cresolis compositus in a pint of warm water may be administered as an intestinal disinfectant.

In case of serious losses from this disease, a veterinarian should be consulted immediately.

Acetonemia (Ketosis or Chronic Milk Fever)

For many years the condition now recognized as acetonemia has been observed in dairy cows during the lactation or milking period. Because of certain nervous symptoms somewhat like those of milk fever, acetonemia was thought to be an a typical form of that disease and has been occasionally referred to as chronic milk fever. The disease is discussed in the article on Nutritional Diseases of Cattle. It might be added here that most uncomplicated cases respond quickly and make a rapid recovery following the administration of one or more treatments with dextrose, the required number varying in different animals. The dosage of dextrose is 500 cubic centimeters of a 40 percent solution given daily, either intravenously (in the veins) or subcutaneously (under the skin) and this treatment may be continued for several days or until there is definite evidence of improvement. Well-marked cases of acetonemia, whether complicated or not, should be treated by a qualified veterinarian.

Pseudorabies (Mad Itch)

Pseudorabies is an infectious disease of cattle characterized by intense pruritis (itching) and paralysis, which usually results in death in 12 to 48 hours. The disease was first described by Aujeszky in Hungary in 1902 and because of symptoms suggestive of rabies, it was designated pseudorabies. The marked evidence of itching in affected animals has led cattle owners in this country to call it mad itch. It is also known as infectious bulbar paralysis and Aujeszky's disease. The disease is now known to be present on both the North and South American Continents, particularly in Brazil and the United States. In this country it has probably existed in the Middle West for a considerable time.

In 1930, Shope (*13*)[2] described an outbreak of mad itch in cattle in Iowa. Subsequent reports of outbreaks in the same State were made by Murray (*11*), Rossing (*12*) and other veterinarians. The disease has also been observed occasionally in other parts of the country.

The mortality rate, in outbreaks of mad itch is quite high; most of the cattle affected die. The economic losses have not been very great, however, owing to the rather limited extent of the infection in this country up to the present.

In his studies of the disease, Shope (*13*) found it to be due to a filtrable virus and in his experimental comparisons of the virus of the disease in this country with that of the European disease he reached a tentative conclusion that the causative agents of the two diseases were probably the same, with certain demonstrable differences in the two strains of viruses.

Recently Morrill and Graham (*10*) reported a spontaneous outbreak of mad itch in a herd of cattle in Illinois. These investigators made some very interesting experimental studies of the disease and reported the isolation from the spinal cord of a steer of a filtrable virus which was indistinguishable from the virus of the European disease.

---

[2] Italic numbers in parentheses refer to Literature Cited.

The virus is most concentrated in the tissue fluids at the point of inoculation and in the brain tissues. In Europe the causative virus has been found with considerable regularity in the blood of affected animals. In the United States Shope found the virus in certain organs such as the lungs and liver of experimental animals, as well as in the brain and certain other tissues, but he found it difficult to demonstrate the virus in the blood.

The natural mode of infection is not definitely known. Available evidence indicates that the disease is not contagious, that is, it is not spread from animal to animal by contact and that infection probably takes place through injury or abrasions of the skin on some part of the body, probably most frequently in the region of the head and neck, though somewhat less frequently the skin lesions are observed on certain parts of the buttocks and thighs. The disease also affects swine, which may become carriers of the infection and are therefore believed to be potential spreaders of the disease among cattle. It is also rather common among rats and it is thought probable that these animals may become carriers. Some observers are of the opinion that the frequent head lesions or injuries, are caused by the bites of infected rats and that it is very probable that domestic animals may be infected in this manner. The fact that the disease is usually limited to certain herds and premises also tends to confirm the opinion that rats are a probable source of infection.

The symptoms vary somewhat in individual cases. Usually there is a marked rise of temperature, which may reach 108° or 109° F. There may be loss of appetite. Among the first symptoms to be noted is increased alertness or nervousness, which is quickly followed by an intense itching, shown by the animals continually licking or rubbing an area of skin on some part of the body–perhaps on the hindquarters or in the region of the head. The licking may become so vigorous as to produce a rasping sound. As the itching becomes more intense, the licking or rubbing of the affected area evidently does not allay the irritation and the animal begins to rub violently against any objects in the vicinity, such as barbed wire or posts and in some cases may even bite or gnaw itself. Some animals may bellow loudly, kick spasmodically with the hind legs and occasionally run violently into objects. There is usually excessive salivation or drooling of saliva from the mouth. As a result of the rubbing and mechanical injury, the skin is denuded of hair and raw, bleeding surfaces are seen. The skin becomes markedly thickened and a fluid may ooze from the area, which eventually becomes a raw, bleeding surface. Occasionally the animal may appear depressed and sleepy. Unsteadiness of gait and possibly paralysis of the hindquarters develop. The affected animals become progressively weaker and death follows in 12 to 48 hours, sometimes preceded by an increasing evidence of paralysis or irregular convulsions, violent tossing of the head, loud groaning and shallow breathing. In occasional cases the animal may not show all the symptoms described and in some instances the intense itching may be entirely absent. In these cases the affected animals may be ill for several days and toward the end have convulsions, drool at the mouth and grind the teeth.

On autopsy the denuded area of skin will be found to be dark, thickened and leathery in appearance and a serous, bloody and sometimes gelatinous fluid is seen infiltrating the tissues under the skin. If the animal has been down for a considerable length of time before death, there may be edema or watery swelling, of the lungs. Occasionally petechiae (pin-point hemorrhages) are seen in the heart and pericardium and the amount of fluid in the heart sac is increased. These heart lesions have led in some instances to confusing the disease with hemorrhagic septicemia. In the central nervous system there may be congestion and small hemorrhages of the meninges or brain coverings. No organic lesions are found on autopsy that can be considered as characteristic or definitely diagnostic of the disease.

The disease may be differentiated from rabies chiefly by its rapid and fatal course and the usual severe itching, which is not in evidence in rabies. Furious attacks and aggressive behavior on the part of affected animals, common in rabies, are seldom seen in pseudorabies and the virus is not found in the saliva, as it is in rabies.

There is no known treatment for the disease and prevention will likewise continue to be a difficult problem until more information is available concerning the means by which animals become infected. When the disease appears in a herd, as a precautionary procedure the healthy cattle should be separated from the sick and removed to different barns or pastures and the quarters occupied by the sick animals should be thoroughly cleaned and disinfected. Hogs should not be permitted to run with the cattle. A campaign of rat extermination would also be of extreme importance on premises where there have been outbreaks of mad itch in cattle.

The More Common Types of Tumors in Cattle

Cattle are subject to a variety of tumors, most of which are of rare occurrence. It is the intention here to consider rather briefly only three of the types that are more frequently encountered, namely, papilloma or common wart; epithelioma, commonly referred to as cancer eye; and a group of internal lymphoid tumors, which are particularly characterized by hyperplasia or enlargement of the various lymph glands of the body.

Papilloma or Common Warts

The common wart, *Verruca vulgaris*, is a specific type of epithelial (skin) overgrowth, nonmalignant in character. Warts are of common occurrence in animals and in man. Adults may be affected by them, but the young are far more susceptible.

Warts on cattle, particularly calves and yearlings, are guite common. They are found on many parts of the body, but their location depends somewhat on the age of the animal. In cows, warts usually occur on the udder or teats, whereas in calves under 1 year of age they are seen most frequently on various parts of the head-on the ears and around the eyes and mouth–and on the sides of the neck and shoulders.

Warts may spread from the original location to different parts of the body and may eventually cover large areas of the skin. Occasionally, particularly on young cattle, they become large and pendulous (Fig. 1) and as a result sap the strength and stunt the growth of the animals. Their chief damage, however, is to calf skins and cattle hides after tanning. The tanned hides have roughened and weak spots where the warts occurred on the skin and they frequently contain numerous pits or holes in places where the skin was thickly studded with warts, as on the shoulders. These defects give a moth–eaten appearance to the finished leather and the parts affected are considered worthless.

The reduction in the value of hides because of warts usually varies from a small percentage to 25 percent and sometimes more, depending on the extent of skin areas affected. Cattle buyers make discounts for warty animals purchased In the markets. Since a considerable number of animals are affected with warts and the hides of many of them are greatly reduced in value, the yearly loss in leather is doubtless large, although no definite figures are available.

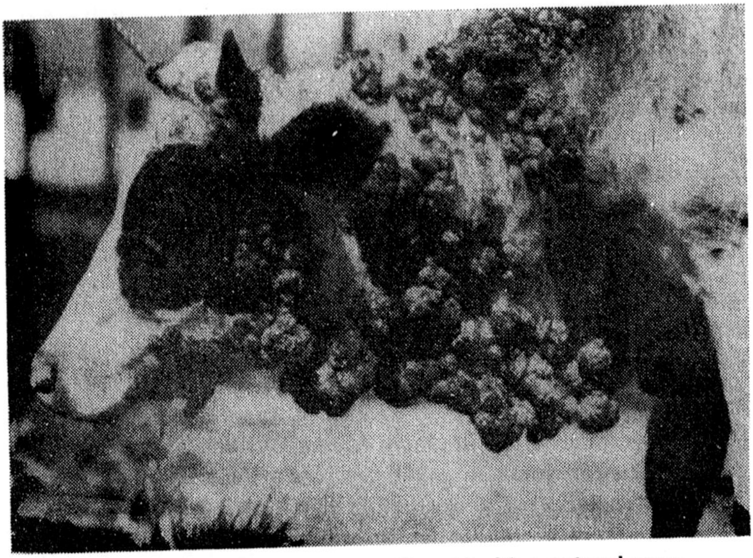

Fig. 1: A heifer about 18 months old with a natural case of common warts.

Warts vary greatly in shape and size. They may be thin, long and club-shaped, an inch or more in length and occur singly or in clusters or they may become large cauliflower like tumors several inches in diameter, in extreme cases weighing several pounds. Occasionally they occur as broad, slightly elevated masses. They may be either hard or soft. The large cauliflower like growths are usually soft and show a tendency to bleed and slough and frequently they give off offensive odors.

Common warts in cattle have been shown by experiments to be infectious. The in fective agent is what is known as a filtrable virus, meaning that it will pass through an earthen, germ-retaining filter. By experimental skin inoculations with wart material, these growths can be produced with a fair degree of regularity in healthy cattle under 1 year of age (Fig. 2). Under ordinary circumstances, infection is thought to take place through injuries to the skin when the injured part comes in contact with warty animals, rubbing posts, fences, buildings or any structure which an affected animal has touched.

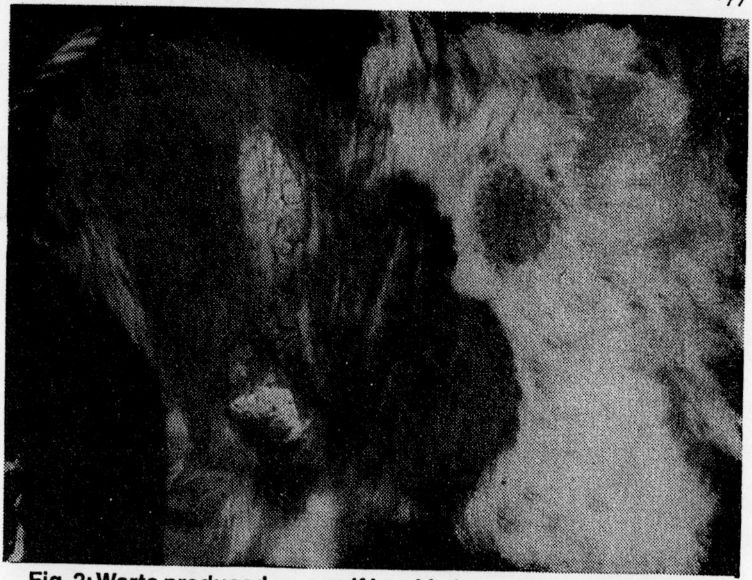

Fig. 2: Warts produced on a calf by skin inoculation with filtered material obtained from the warts on the heifer shown in figure 1.

Treatment and Prevention

Warts occasionally disappear without treatment of any kind, especially as animals become older. Most cases, however, require definite and systematic treatment.

Warts that are small at the place of attachment may be removed by either clipping them off with sterile scissors or tying a sterile thread or slender cord tightly around the wart near the base so that it will slough off in a few days. The stumps of the warts should be touched with either glacial acetic acid or tincture of iodine. Tying off is recommended also for warts which because of their size are likely to contain a number of blood vessels that would bleed if the warts were removed by cutting. The roots or bases of such warts also should be treated with glacial acetic acid or sliver nitrate. The removal of extremely large warts by surgical means should be performed by a veterinarian. Before warts become excessively large they may be destroyed by daily applications of glacial acetic acid or tincture of iodine. Before applying acetic acid, protect the healthy skin immediately surrounding the warts by thoroughly greasing with petrolatum or lard, taking care not to grease the warts since that would protect them also from the acid. Small warts, such as those oil the udders of Cows, will sometimes disappear if kept soft by daily applications of sweet oil or castor oil.

If warts are numerous and cover large areas of the body, it may be advisable to give internal treatment also. The usual internal treatment for various skin disorders, including warts, is arsenic in the form of Fowler's solution. The dose is 1 tablespoonful twice daily for cattle 6 to 12 months of age. This method, however, should be considered only an indirect treatment and it should be used only under the supervision of a veterinarian. Since arsenic may pass into the milk, Fowler's solution should not be given to milking cows.

A wart vaccine is now being used to some extent, with reports of rather favorable results. The treatment is still in the experimental stage, however and further observations will be required to determine its efficacy.

Preventive measures consist in removing all warty cattle, particularly calves and yearlings, from the herd and cleaning and disinfecting all exposed stables, pens, chutes and rubbing posts. In dairy herds, cows with warts on their teats and udders should be milked last and the milkers should be careful to wash and disinfect their hands thoroughly after each milking to prevent the possible spread of the virus from one animal to another. The essential point to keep in mind is that these growths are infectious or catching.

Epithelioma (Carcinoma or Cancer Eye)

Epithelioma of the eyes of cattle, more commonly referred to as cancer eye, is a cancerous or malignant type of tumor which primarily attacks the eye or related tissues. This eye tumor appears to be somewhat more prevalent in the West and Southwest than elsewhere in the United States, although it may be seen in all parts of the country.

As in the case of other malignant tumors, the specific cause of epithelioma of the eyes of cattle is not known. A number of possible contributing causes have been suggested, such as irritation of the eyes by dust sand, insects or other irritants. The strong rays of the sun also have been mentioned as a possible cause, particularly in the case of the Hereford breed of cattle, which appears to be particularly susceptible, to caner eye. The theory is that the lack of protective pigment or coloring matter, in the eye membranes and skin surrounding the eyes in this breed results in a sensitization of the tissues to sunlight and the irritation thus set up may lead to the cancerous condition. While it seems logical that irritation may play some part as a causative factor in cancer eye, nothing of a specific nature has been definitely proved.

The growth may have its origin in the membrana nictitans, at the inner canthus or angle, of the eye, in the mucous lining of the lids or in the front part or cornea, of the eyeball. It may appear at first as a small reddish mass with a tendency as it becomes larger to assume a fungus like or papillary (nipplelike) appearance. Such growths are very sensitive and susceptible to injury and when injured bleed freely. The eye proper is not usually affected in the early stages, but eventually it becomes involved and the sight is destroyed. The tumorous mass usually becomes infected with bacteria, a condition that is followed by suppuration or pus formation and extensive destruction of tissues, accompanied by a very foul odor. In the warm months it is not unusual to see these eye growth infested by the larvae or maggots, of the screwworm fly. The eye is eventually completely destroyed by the growth, which then spreads to the surrounding tissues, involving both the soft structures and the bone of the orbit (Fig. 3). As the growth becomes more extensive, the bones of the nose and head may be affected.

In the more advanced or long-standing cases, the cancerous cells are disseminated through metastasis or transference to other tissues and organs, chiefly by way of the lymph stream. The parotid lymph gland, which lies in rather close proximity to the eye, soon becomes involved and the growth may spread to other lymph glands of the head and neck regions through lymph drainage. By the same means of distribution or metastasis, the lungs may become involved and in some cases the liver and other organs.

In all advanced cases of cancer eye there is a drain on the animal's vitality. There may be absorption of toxins from the infected tumor, resulting in decline in general condition and emaciation. Cattle owners should always bear in mind that epithelioma of the eye is definitely cancerous or malignant, in all cases and eventually will spread to other tissues and cause the death of the animal unless this is prevented through early operative procedure.

Little can be done to alleviate the condition after the tumor has become extensive enough to involve the entire eye and adjacent

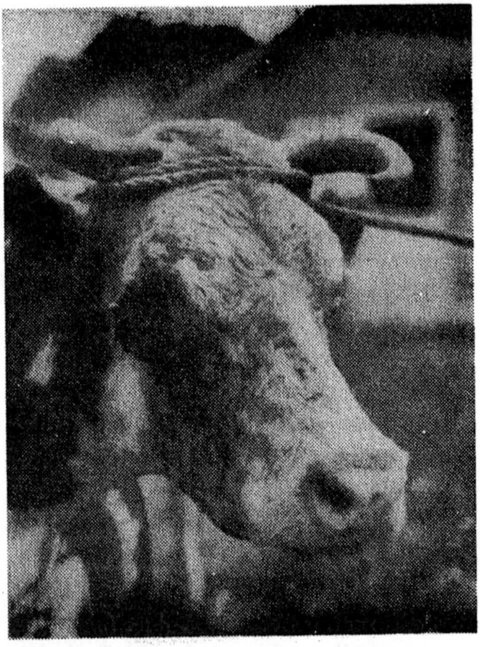

Fig. 3: Epithelioma or cancer eye, in a cow, Note that the eye is completely destroyed and that the growth involves the surrounding tissues.

tissues. In such cases, if the animal is still in fair condition, it should be sent to market for slaughter, subject to inspection. Under Federal meat-inspection regulations, if the tumor is still localized or confined largely to the eye structures and has not involved the lymph glands, the head is condemned and the remainder of the carcass passed for food.

Operative procedure consists in the total removal of the cancerous tissue, together with removal (enucleation) of the eyeball, which is likely to be involved after the growth is well established. It is extremely important that the operation be performed as soon as a definite diagnosis of cancer eye has been made. When it has been performed early enough, the results have usually been quite satisfactory. Needless to say, such operations should be performed by a veterinarian who is thoroughly skilled and fully equipped to carry out the necessary technical procedure.

Lymphocytoma, Lymphatic Leukemia and Pseudoleukemia

There is a third group of tumors of rather common occurrence in cattle which are lymphoid in nature–that is, they primarily affect the lymphoid tissue and the lymph glands in particular, which usually show marked hyperplasia or enlargement. These internal neoplasms or morbid growths, are malignant in character and have been referred to by pathologists as lymphoma, lymphocytoma, lymphosarcoma, lymphatic leukemia, pseudoleukemia and by various other designations. While there is a marked resemblance in the gross appearance of all the conditions designated by these names and also in the microscopical appearance in many instances, occasional slight differences are seen in the cell structure and this accounts for the variation in terminology. There is still much confusion regarding the proper classification of these lymphoid conditions–whether they should be classified as several distinct varieties of new growths or be placed in a single group.[3]

One of the first indications of the disease usually observed is a noticeable enlargement of the superficial lymph glands (those near the surface), particularly the submaxillary gland, situated in the region of the throat, the prescapular gland, Just in front of the shoulder and the precrural gland, in the flank region (Fig. 4). The supramammary lymph gland, which is above and behind the udder, may also be enlarged. As a result of metastasis or dissemination of the tumor material to other tissues and organs, there may be evidences of general disturbance such as irregular heart action, difficult breathing, general weakness and progressive emaciation. In the later stages there is loss of appetite, extreme weakness and finally death. These lymphoid conditions are usually chronic and terminate in death in a number of weeks to several months after the first evidence of the disease is noted.

---

[3] Feldman (*7*) places these lymphoid tumors in the general class of lymphoblastoma. While there is a persistent similarity In most of these new growths, certain exceptions are encountered In which there are rather definite variations. One such exception is found in cases of true leukemia, in which there is a definite change in the ratio of blood cells or a marked increase in the white blood corpuscles. These cases are rather rare (*4*). Another definite deviation from the usual type has been reported more recently by Bengston (*2*) of the Bureau of Animal Industry. This type was found to be more definitely sarcomatous in nature, and he designated it as reticulum sarcoma.

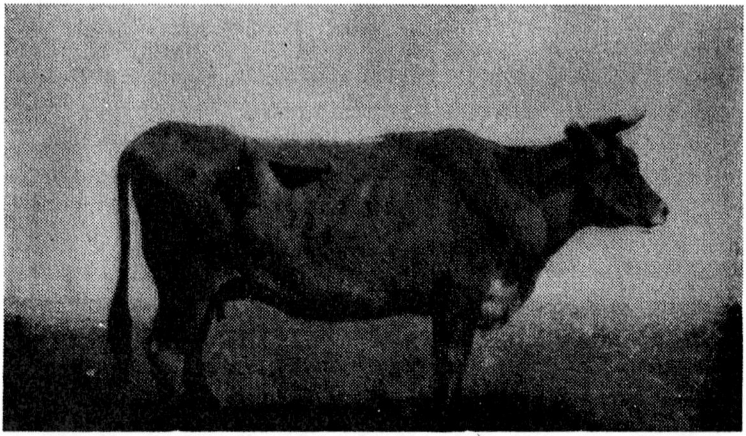

Fig. 4: A cow with lymphatic leukemia. Note the greatly enlarged lymph glands-the prescapular, in front of the shoulder, and the precrural, in the flank region.

On autopsy the lymph glands will be found greatly enlarged. There is usually an edematous or watery condition of the various tissues. When the disease has extended to the different organs, there may be marked enlargement of the spleen and light or grayish areas of spots may be seen in the tissue of the heart, liver and kidney. Occasionally growths may be seen in the stomachs and in cows the uterus may be affected. Nodular tumor growths are found in the body cavities in some cases.

It may sometimes be necessary to differentiate the lymphoid conditions from certain other diseases in which the lymph glands become enlarged, such as tuberculosis and actinomycosis (described later in this same article). The possibility of tuberculosis may be eliminated through the tuberculin test and examinations for actinomycosis or other infectious conditions may be made through a biopsy or removal from the living animal by surgery of a portion of an enlarged gland for laboratory examination, culturing, etc. Blood examinations are also valuable aids in diagnosing leukemia.

There are no known methods of treatment or prevention of these lymphoid conditions, which are fatal to all animals affected.

Actinomycosis and Actinobacillosis

For many years most of the tumorlike swellings or enlargements of the tissues of the head and throat in cattle, commonly referred to as lumpy jaw, big jaw and wooden tongue, were diagnosed as actinomycosis. It is now known that there is another infectious condition, technically referred to as actinobacillosis, particularly involving the soft tissues, in which the tissue changes are very similar to those in actinomycosis. The two diseases are due to entirely different types of micro-organisms, the causative agent in actinomycosis being *Actinomyces bovis*, the ray fungus and in actinobacillosis, *Actinobacilus lignieresi*. Frequently certain types of pyogenic or pusproducing, bacteria are also associated with these infections.

Actinomycosis and actinobacillosis are both chronic infectious diseases and the former tendency to confuse them or consider them as one disease was due largely to the marked similarity of the lesions or tissue changes and also possibly to the fact that the causative organisms, as seen microscopically in pus preparations and sections from the affected tissues, have a similar club formation and rosette arrangement. It seems logical, therefore, to consider the two types together and at the same time to indicate any specific points of difference between them.

Brief descriptions of the microscopic findings and also of certain details disclosed by autopsy, are given at the end of this section, Actinomycosis and actinobacillosis affect cattle in all parts of the United States, possibly being somewhat more prevalent in the West than elsewhere. Fatalities are comparatively few and the diseases are ordinarily not considered of great economic importance. The records of the Federal meat-inspection service indicate, however, that these infections are responsible for considerable losses every year from condemnation of affected carcasses and parts of carcasses.

The infective organisms are widespread in nature and gain entrance to the tissues most frequently through injuries or abrasions of the mucous membranes of the mouth cavity and throat region. It has been assumed that Actinomyees or the ray fungus, is present on grasses and grains and that the sharp awns of grains and certain grasses, such as foxtail, are the means by which the organisms are introduced into the deeper tissues of the mouth through the mucous membrane. The gums of cattle are very sensitive and more or less lacerated during the teething period and in all probability this affords a means of entrance for such infections in many cases, since actinomycotic infections are seen most frequently in young cattle during the period of changing teeth.

Some observers are of the opinion that the mouth may be the chief normal habitat of these organisms and that they invade the tissues and produce disease only under unusual conditions or following irritation and injuries to the mucous membranes. In areas in the Southwest where the fruit of the cactus is eaten by cattle, it is thought probable that many cases of actinomycotic infection are due to injures of the mucous membrane of the mouth by the small cactus spines or spicules.

Lesions of Actinomycosis

Actinomycosis may occur in the soft tissues but as a rule is confined to the bones of the head, particularly the maxillae or jawbones, the lower jawbone being most frequently involved. The nasal bones are occasionally involved when the upper jaw is affected and this may result in difficult breathing. The bone lesions produced are those of a rarefying ostitis–that is, the bone becomes enlarged and rarefied or spongy. The small cavities in the spongy bone are filled with pus. The palate and gums adjacent to the involved bone become swollen and inflamed and the teeth may become loosened. The bony growth may extend outward through the soft tissues and skin, eventually appearing on the external surface as a mass of granulation tissue or funguslike growths, with a foul odor. The infection may also extend inward, resulting in similar lesions, cauliflower like masses of inflamed tissue containing openings or cavities which discharge a sticky yellowish or creamy pus in which can be seen very minute, pale yellow grains, the so-called sulfur granules characteristic of this type of infection.

Lesions of Actinobacillosis

So far as is known at the present time, the lesions of actinobacillosis are confined to the soft tissues. In the tissues of the head or cervical (neck) region, the lesions are characterized by movable swellings; or tumefactions, under the skin, varying from the size of a walnut to that of an egg or larger. The lymph glands of the cervical region may be involved and much enlarged. The consistency of the tumor formations may vary somewhat in the different tissues, the firmness of the growth depending on the amount of fibrous connective tissue present. These abscessed enlargements eventually break through the skin, discharging a creamy pus. Frequently the opening or discharging cavity becomes filled with reddish granulomatous (funguslike) tissue.

The tongue is often involved in actinobacillosis and there may or may not be ulceration. The ulcers most frequently have their beginning at the transverse depression or so-called groove, on the upper surface of the tongue. They usually show as round or oval depressed areas with elevated, irregular and ragged edges. The ulcerations are frequently covered with debris such as hairs and vegetable matter and there is usually a foul odor.

Sometimes when the tongue is involved there may also be ulcerations of the mucous membrane and abscess formation in the region of the pharynx, larynx and trachea. The lymph glands of the throat region may also be affected. When the tongue is extensively involved in the chronic inflammatory process, there is a very marked increase in the fibrous tissue of the organ (fibrosis) and as a result the tongue becomes increasingly hard and immobile and may protrude from the mouth; this condition has given rise to the term "wooden tongue." The tongue is manipulated with great difficulty and there is almost constant drooling of saliva. Eventually there is practically a complete loss of pretension or ability to take feed into the mouth, mastication is seriously interfered with, the animal becomes weak and greatly emaciated and it may die of exhaustion.

Lesions in the pharynx may take the form of mushroom like growths or pendulous masses, which in some cases may completely fill the pharyngeal cavity, seriously interfering with swallowing and breathing.

In addition to the external lesions described, there may also be a distribution of the infection to various internal organs and tissues, including the lungs, liver, kidneys, spleen, brain, mammary gland, testes, urinary bladder, muscles and serous linings of the body cavities. Cases in which the skin and subcutaneous tissues of different parts of the body and the extremities were infected have also been reported.

Infection of the peritoneum–the membrane lining the cavity of the abdomen–is not uncommon in cattle and three such cases were re- ported by Creech (3) some years ago in calves approximately 8 weeks old. Owing to the age of the animals, these were unusually interesting cases. No other lesions were found and the portal of entry of the infective agent was not determined.

Symptoms, Prevention and Treatment

The course of both of these diseases is always slow or chronic in character, extending over a period of months or even several years. The general effects depend largely on the location of the lesions and their interference with the natural functions of the body. For example, when the jawbones are involved, there may be loss of teeth and consequent interference with chewing. Growths in the pharynx may inhibit swallowing and cause difficult breathing or partial suffocation. The difficulties caused by involvement of the tongue, particularly in the more marked cases of wooden tongue, have already been mentioned. Such interference with the body functions naturally leads to depletion and emaciation. Otherwise, localized lesions do not seem definitely to affect the general health of the diseased animals.

Prevention of actinomycosis and actinobacillosis is somewhat difficult in the absence of definite knowledge as to how animals contract these diseases. Available information indicates that they are probably infectious rather than contagious in character. It has been found extremely difficult to transmit actinomycosis by experimental inoculation, but less difficulty has been experienced in transmitting actinobacillosis. While there is little evidence to indicate that the infections are directly transmissible from animal to animal, either actinomycosis or actinobacillosis may affect large groups of animals in the same herd. This suggests that if the disease is not contagious, all the animals contracted it from the same source, possibly the feed. Regardless of the mode of infection, animals with lesions from which discharging pus may contaminate the food or surrounding objects should not be permitted to remain in pastures or feed lots with healthy cattle.

Treatment of actinomycosis is not very satisfactory, largely because of the nature of the lesions involving the bone tissues, but actinobacillosis yields quite readily to treatment in most cases. The most satisfactory treatment is to give, iodine, usually in the form of sodium or potassium iodide, in doses of 1½ to 2½ drams daily, dissolved in water and administered as a drench. When there are lesions of the tongue or pharynx, care must be used to see that none of the drug reaches the lungs, as this may cause pneumonia. After a week or 10 days, the treated animals may show indications of the cumulative effect of the drug or iodism, evidenced by a flow of tears, catarrh of the nose, loss of appetite and scurfy skin. When such symptoms appear, treatments should be discontinued for a few days or a week, after which they may be resumed. Definite curative results may be expected to appear in 2 to 6 weeks, the length of time varying in different cases. Some cases do not respond to the treatment and if no definite evidence of improvement is seen after 3 or 4 weeks, the treatment should be discontinued. It is inadvisable to administer potassium iodide to cows that are lactating, as the drug is secreted in the milk and also tends to reduce the amount. Also the drug should not be given to cows in advanced pregnancy, as it may cause abortion.

Tincture of iodine may be applied externally to the enlargements or Lugol's solution of iodine may be injected in the region of the swellings. The large cutaneous tumors may be incised, the contents or necrotic material, removed and the incision packed with gauze saturated with tincture of iodine.

Surgery would be indicated in some cases, particularly when the tumor formations are so situated that removal may be readily accomplished.

In these diseases it is always advisable to consult a veterinarian and be guided by his opinion as to the required method of treatment in each individual case. A veterinarian's services should, of course, be obtained in all cases in which surgery is indicated.

While some cases of slight actinomycotic infection of the bone may yield to the iodine treatment, it will usually prove more economical to flatten animals so affected for slaughter.

Since man is susceptible to both actinomycosis and actinobacillosis, animals with these diseases sent to market for slaughter ought always to be inspected by a veterinarian in order to determine the suitability of the carcasses for food.

The Federal meat-inspection regulations require the condemnation of the entire carcasses of cattle showing generalized lesions of actinomycosis or actinobacillosis. If the carcasses of affected animals otherwise show a well-nourished condition and the lesions are strictly realized in certain tissues of the body, they may be passed for food after the removal and condemnation of the parts or organs affected. When the head and tongue are affected, both must be condemned. In cases in which the lesions of the jaw are very slight and strictly localized, with no indications whatever of extension of infection to the surrounding and related tissues, the tongue, if entirely free from the disease, may be passed for food.

Findings on Microscopic Examination and Autopsy

Microscopically as well as in visible details, the lesions of actinomycosis and actinobacillosis as seen in tissue sections are very similar, consisting of granulation tissue composed of lymphoid and epithelioid cells and usually numbers of giant cells, with centers of focal necrosis and possibly some calcification. In the degenerated areas will be seen heavy infiltrations of polymorphonucleal leucocytes–the most common type of white blood cells–and some plasma cells. The cellular tissue is surrounded by zones of fibrous tissue.

Within the meshwork of the fibrous formations in actinobacillosis are small cavities or pockets filled with cellular elements or puslike material in which can be seen small yellowish granules similar to those described in actinomycosis. These are the colonies of organisms. If the small granules are examined under the microscope either in press preparations from the pus or in tissue sections, they will be seen as rounded masses with club-shaped radiations that give them a rosette appearance. In most respects the appearance of the rosettes in both types of infection is quite similar with ordinary staining, but with special staining, as with Gram stain, the actinomyces give positive results or retain the stain, while the actinobacilli give negative results or fail to retain the stain. In the former, fungus mycelia may be seen, while in the latter only bacteria or bacilli are present. As a rule the rosettes are larger in actinomycosis than in actinobacillosis.

Affected tongue foci on sectioning, will be seen to contain yellowish, sticky, puslike material. Nodular formations or small lumps and fistulous (tubelike) tracts or cavities may be seen in the muscular substance of the tongue in some cases.

In the lungs the disease is manifested as grayish or grayish-yellow nodular masses which contain a thick puslike material and fragments of tissue (detritus). In some cases the lesions may be seen as grayish, soft. moist areas. On sectioning the affected lung tissue, the yellowish grains or sulfur granules, previously referred to, may be seen distributed through the lesions, which aids in differentiating this type of infection from tuberculosis. In advanced cases the lesions, may assume the form of soft, grayish-yellow masses, enclosed in a membrane and several inches in diameter, in which portions of the affected tissue may be broken down or semifluid. The lymph glands associated with the lungs may also be affected.

Somewhat similar lesions are found in the liver and other organs, the general character of the tissue changes depending somewhat on the amount of connective tissue present and the extent of necrosis and disintegration of the tissues affected.

Nasal Granuloma (Snoring Disease)

Nasal granuloma, as the name indicates, is a disease of the nasal cavities of cattle in which there is thickening of the nasal mucous lining. The condition causes more or less interference with the passage of air in breathing, resulting in a peculiar snoring sound; hence the more common name snoring disease.

Nasal granuloma has existed among the cattle of India for a long time, but it had not been observed in any other country until a similar disease was reported in 1933 to be present in the United States (*5*). The disease was first discovered in this country in a dairy herd at the Iberia Livestock Experiment Station, at Jeanerette, La. It had apparently existed in this herd for 4 or 5 years prior to the time studies made of the disease were reported. Subsequently the disease has been observed in several other herds in Louisiana but apparently has not been definitely recognized in any other part of the country.

While there may be a loss of general condition in affected animals in the more advanced stages of the disease, so far as is known, fatalities seldom occur. Since the disease is also very limited in extent, it may be considered of minor economic Importance at the present time.

Nasal granuloma occurs in India in two forms. One is parasitic in nature, being caused by a schistosome worm or fluke, while the other form is caused by a sporozoan organism (one that reproduces by means of spores) of the genus *Rhinosporidium*. The specific cause of the disease in the United States has not been definitely determined.

Bacteriological studies examinations for the presence of parasites have thus far given entirely negative results. Experimental animal inoculations have likewise failed to yield any specific information with regard to the cause of the disease.

The first symptoms usually noticed are sneezing and nasal discharge of a mucopurulent material–a mixture of mucus and pus (Fig. 5). In the more acute cases this material is frequently mixed with blood and may also contain small portions of destroyed mucous membrane. The bloody discharges may be seen on the stable floor or on the grass or ground where the affected animals have been pastured.

As the disease progresses, difficult breathing is noticed and a peculiar droning sound or snoring, can be heard for some distance. The affected cattle show a characteristic wrinkling of the skin surrounding the wing of the nostril, resulting from the extra effort

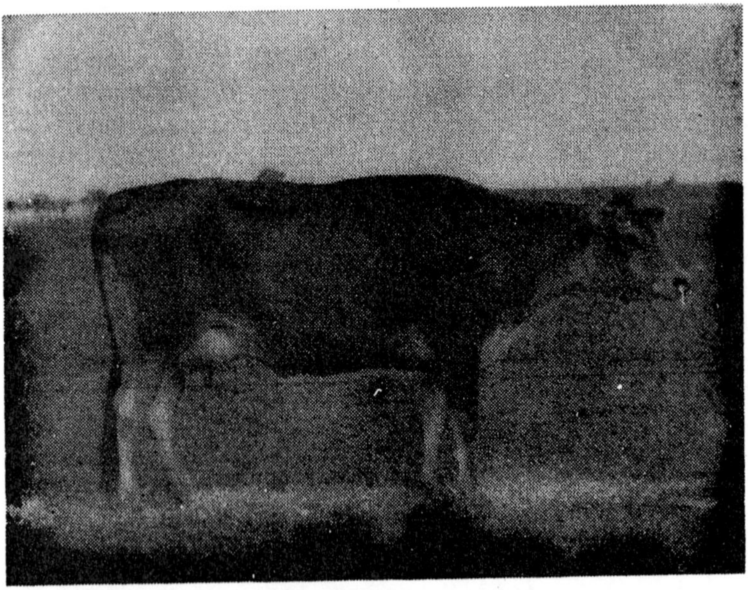

Fig. 5: Cow first found to be affected with nasal granuloma at the Iberia Livestock Experiment Station. Note the characteristic expansion of the nostril and the nasal discharge.

required in breathing because of the partial closing or obstruction. of the nasal cavity. The difficult breathing is more pronounced during the worm months and the disease tends to subside of becomes more or less dormant during the cool season.

Certain treatments for this disease have been tried without very marked success. None have given permanent relief and further experimentation is probably required to find a satisfactory or specific treatment.

The lesions or tissue changes are confined strictly to the nasal mucous membrane and rarely extend beyond the first 3 inches of the anterior nares or nostrils. The lesions may extend entirely around the nasal. cavity, including the mucosa of the nasal septum or wall separating the nostrils.

In the more acute cases the mucosa becomes markedly congested and this is followed by hemorrhages and sloughing, leaving small denuded areas from which blood or a mixture of blood and mucus escapes from time to time. In addition to the more acute changes the nasal mucosa becomes thickly studded with numerous small, grayish, tubercle like nodules varying in size (Fig. 6). In cases of long duration there is marked thickening of the nasal mucosa, due to the extensive chronic fibrous changes.

Histological Changes

While the histological changes are essentially those characteristic of granulation tissue, the lesions vary somewhat with the stage of the disease.

In the newer nodules the invading cells are chiefly round or migratory, cells and leucocytes. As the disease progresses, fibroblasts become more evident and groups or masses of eosinophile cells are seen distributed through the newly formed fibrous structure. Finally in the chronic stage the entire affected portion of the mucosa may undergo fibrosis. Certain other changes, such as perivascular infiltration, endarteritis, degeneration and vacuolization of the mucous glands, have also been noted. Few well-formed giant cells have been observed in sections.

In occasional sections made from the more acute nodular lesions a limited number of small round bodies, fairly definite in outline, have appeared. Some of these showed slightly serrated borders and a number of the bodies seemed to be nucleated. Some were also

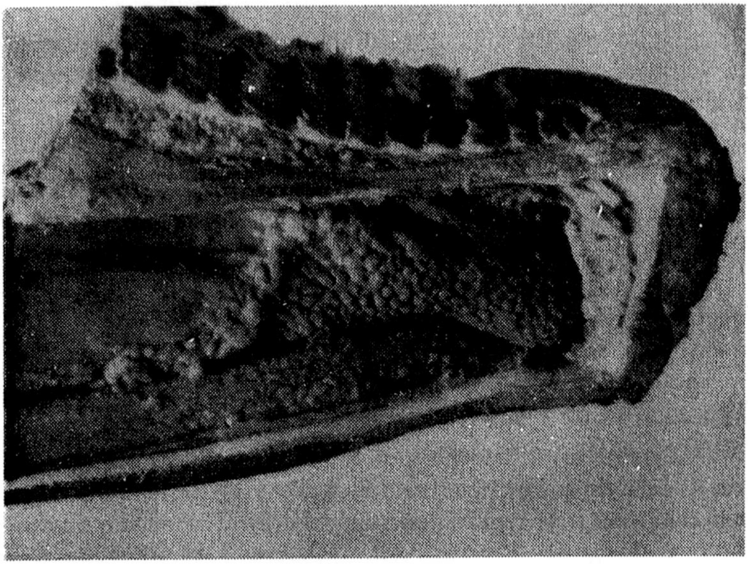

Fig. 6: Nodular lesions in the nasal cavity of a cow affected with nasal granuloma.

surrounded by a brownish-pigmented circle or capsule. Small bodies which were thought to be similar in character also have been found in fresh preparations of the nodular material. Dikmans (*6*) observed similar small bodies in his studies of the disease and expressed the opinion that they probably had an etiological relation to the disease and possibly were related to the genus *Rhinosporidium.*

Goiter

Goiter is characterized by enlargement of the thyroid glands, which are situated in the region of the throat. While it, may occur in adult cattle in the goiter districts, the general health of such animals does not appeared to be impaired (*8*). The chief significance of goiter in cattle and other animals is as a disease of the newborn.

Specific Ophthalmia (Infectious Conjuctivities Infectious Kertitis or Pinkeye)

Inflammatory conditions of the eyes of cattle are referred to medically as ophthalmia, conjunctivitis and keratitis, the term used depending somewhat on the parts of the eye involved or the extent of the inflammation. The common name for all of these is pinkeye. Most frequently these inflammatory conditions have their beginning as a conjunctivitis or inflammation of the conjunctiva, which is the lining membrane of the eyelids and also covers the visible part of the eyeball. When the inflammation becomes more extensive and involves the deeper structures of the cornea–the front or transparent portion of the eye–the condition is referred to as keratitis.

The disease is quite widespread throughout the country. As with other diseases of an enzootic nature (that is, prevalent in various districts), it is difficult to explain why it becomes more widespread and virulent during certain years and in certain localities. Whether seasonal and environmental conditions may influence such outbreaks is not definitely known. Although it is apparently not confined to any particular season, the disease is rarely observed during the winter months. It affects old and young animals alike.

There are practically no fatalities from the disease, but it has an economic aspect because it results in poor condition, loss of body weight, reduction in milk secretion and general lowering of production when a large number of animals are affected.

Available evidence as obtained from outbreaks in certain herds indicates that these marked inflammatory conditions of the eyes of cattle are infectious in nature, but it is also very probable that certain predisposing factors play a rather important part–for example, dust, pollen, strong sunlight and irritation or injury caused by insects or by contact with grasses, weeds, stubble, etc. Any irritation or injury makes the eye tissues more susceptible to infection.

A number of different types of bacteria have been found to be associated with the disease, more particularly the pyogenic or pus-producing group of organisms such as staphylococci, streptococci and pyogenic bacilli. The hay bacillus (*Bacillus subtilis*) and organisms of the hemorrhagic septicemia group have been mentioned as possible causes. It has been difficult, however, to incriminate any particularly organism as the specific causative agent.

As evidence of the infectious nature of the disease, the Kansas State Agricultural Experiment Station (9) reported the experimental transmission of keratitis by the inoculation of the eyes of susceptible calves with lachrymal secretions or discharges from the eyes of diseased calves. The inoculated calves developed the eye disease after an incubation period of 3 to 18 days. Filtered eye secretions from affected calves failed to produce the disease in susceptible animals (the use of bacteria-retaining filters would remove any bacteria present). These investigators also isolated a number of different types of bacteria from the diseased eyes of calves, but they were apparently unable to related anyone organism definitely to the disease.

According to further observations of the Kansas investigators, one attack of the disease does not confer immunity. Affected calves held in dark stalls recovered without treatment after 3 to 4 weeks in the disease had not advanced to the point of ulceration of the cornea.

Among the first symptoms observed are a flow of tears and avoidance of light or a tendency to keep the eyes closed. Severe conjunctivitis or reddening of the conjunctiva develops. The eyelids become swollen, hot and sensitive to the touch. The lachrymal discharge from the eyes soon becomes mixed with pus and may be streaked with blood. The skin of the face becomes soiled by the constant discharge from the eyes. As the inflammation progresses, there is involvement of the deeper structures of the eye, particularly the cornea. There is an early cloudiness or opacity of the cornea, which may also be covered by an inflammatory deposit and eventually corneal ulcers (ulcerative keratitis). There may be spontaneous recovery in some cases in which the inflammatory changes are not too far advanced, while in others the disease may become more deep-seated. In the more advanced cases there may be abscess formation of the cornea and possibly in the anterior chamber of the eye. Perforation of the cornea may occur with consequent loss of sight. In extreme cases there may be practically complete destruction of the eye.

There is usually some general disturbance, as evidenced by a rise of temperature, partial loss of appetite, suspended rumination, decrease in the milk secretion and indications of increasing debility in advanced cases.

Prevention and treatment will probably remain more or less unsatisfactory until more definite information is available concerning the specific or primary cause of the condition. It is definitely known, however, as previously indicated, that a number of different types of organisms are associated with the disease and are capable of causing much damage once they have gained entrance to the tissues of the eye. Whether such bacteria are primary causative factors or secondary invaders, it is extremely important that prompt steps be taken for early treatment of the infectious condition in order to prevent possible permanent damage to the eyes or loss of sight.

Treatment

In view of the probably infectious nature of the disease, when the eye affection appears in the herd all unaffected cattle should be moved promptly to other barns or pastures if this is feasible. The diseased cattle should be housed in dark stables or sheds and provided with plenty of fresh drinking water and soft, succulent feed. Depending on the size of the animal, administer 1 to 1½ pounds of Epsom salts dissolved in water.

Cocaine may be applied to the eyes when there is evidence of pain. A 1 percent solution of silver nitrate has given very good results as an eye lotion. This is applied every other day until there are definite indications of improvement, then every third or fourth day until the inflammation subsides. The sliver nitrate solution should be fresh when used and may be applied to the eyes with a soft cotton swab, care being taken not to cause further irritation by undue rubbing or pressure. Less satisfactory results are obtained from applications of boracic acid solution. A more recent treatment recommended for keratitis is mercurochrome. Bardens (*1*) reported having obtained very satisfactory results with mercurochrome in 1- to 4-percent solutions dropped in the eyes several times daily. The stronger solution is recommended in cases of ulceration of the cornea. It is claimed to be less irritating to the eyes than the silver preparations.

Bardens also gives considerable credit to the mixed bacterins for keratitis, used simultaneously with the local mercurochrome treatment. The initial dose of the bacterin was 10 cubic centimeters, increased by 5 to 10 cubic centimeters daily until a maximum of 20 was reached. He found that two doses of bacterin were usually sufficient to correct the condition in dairy cattle.

It appears to be the consensus of opinion among veterinarians that more satisfactory results are obtained in the treatment of the disease when the mixed keratitis bacterins are used in conjunction with local treatments with the mercurochrome or silver nitrate solutions.

The treatments suggested, particularly the bacterin treatments, should be administered by a veterinarian and as in other infectious or contagious diseases, when an outbreak of pinkeye occurs in a herd the owner should promptly consult his local veterinarian and follow his instructions with regard to the best procedure for the eradication of the disease from the herd.

Calf Diphtheria

Calf diphtheria is an acute infectious disease of suckling calves characterized by the formation of a diphtheritic false membrane on the mucous lining of the mouth and pharynx (throat). The disease is confined largely to young suckling calves, sometimes attacking them as early as the third or fourth day after birth, although in severe outbreaks mature animals may become affected. The mortality from the disease is very high. Calf diphtheria is also known as necrotic stomatitis, gangrenous stomatitis, ulcerative stomatitis, necrotic laryngitis, malignant stomatitis and sore mouth.

The disease is caused by a specific organism, *Actinomyces necrophorus*, which is widespread in nature. The organism is strictly anaerobic; that is, it grows only in the absence of oxygen. It gains entrance through wounds in the mucous membrane or lining, of the mouth. Such injuries are usually caused by sharp-pointed particles of food or other objects. Infection may also occur during the eruption of the first teeth after birth. The parts of the mouth most often affected at the beginning of the disease are the base or side of the tongue, the inside of the cheeks adjacent to the molar teeth and the lips. If the infection persists, however, the lesions or tissue injuries, may spread to the hard palate, the gums, the pharynx, the nasal passages, the trachea (windpipe) and the lungs.

Occasionally only one or two animals in a herd may be affected, but in other instances as many as 10 percent may show evidence of the disease.

The first symptoms appear 3 to 5 days after the causative organism gains entrance to the tissues. The affected animal appears depressed and even suckling calves will refuse feed. Drooling of saliva and swallowing movements may be noted. At times a swelling may be observed on the side of the cheek or in the region of the throat. The animal becomes weak and loses flesh rapidly. Where the lesions have become extensive, involving the larynx and nasal passages, there are wheezing, coughing and labored breathing. A sticky, yellowish to greenish-yellow discharge from the nostrils may also be noticed. At this stage of the disease the animal is greatly depressed, extremely weak and emaciated and lies down continuously. Slobbering is profuse and the tongue is swollen and sometimes protrudes from the mouth, which has a very offensive odor.

Soon after gaining entrance to the tissues of the mouth the causative organism multiplies rapidly and a poisonous substance or toxin, is elaborated. This toxin destroys the invaded tissues, resulting in extensive ulceration of the mucous lining of the mouth cavity. In the mouth of an affected animal there may be one or more ulcers on the mucosa of the cheek, on the base of the tongue or along the sides of the tongue. The destroyed tissue has a grayish-yellow appearance and around the borders of the ulcer the tissue will be slightly raised, reddened and granulated in appearance. An exudation or discharge, of albuminous material from the ulcerated areas combines with the dead cellular elements to form a fibrinous mass or membrane, that gradually becomes dry, friable (crumbly) and cheesy. This degenerated tissue sticks tightly and can be scraped or peeled off only with difficulty.

As the disease process spreads, the lesions may involve the deeper tissue structures to a depth of an inch or more. Usually in these cases, there is no tendency toward spontaneous healing and the untreated lesions continue to spread and involve very large areas of the mouth, tongue, larynx (upper part of the windpipe), pharynx and nasal cavities. In cases of long standing the infection becomes more or less generalized and lesions may be found in the lungs, stomach, intestines and liver. In the very acute form of the disease, the animal may die within a week. The cause of death is toxemia or blood poisoning, resulting from the infection rather than the local effects of the disease. In less acute outbreaks, affected animals may live a number of weeks and show extensive lesions.

In mild cases, if the sick animals are given prompt attention in the early stages, treatment may bring about recovery. On the other hand, in the highly virulent outbreaks in which there is extensive involvement of the tissues, treatment is of little avail.

Prevention is of the greatest importance and consists in segregating the sick from the healthy animals, thoroughly cleaning and disinfecting the stables and sheds and carefully examining the healthy animals each day for immediate detection of new cases, which should be isolated as soon as they are found.

Treatment consists in removing the dead tissue from the affected areas and painting the ulcerated surfaces with appropriate medicinal agents, such as a 5-percent solution of potassium permanganate or tincture of iodine. The mouth of an affected calf should be washed frequently with warm water. The strength of the animal should be maintained by feeding nutritious food, such as eggs and milk. As other serious animal diseases, it is advisable to obtain the services of a veterinarian and follow his directions regarding preventive measures and treatment.

Pneumonia

Pneumonia is an inflammation of the lungs in which the air sacs fill up with an inflammatory exudate or discharge. As a result, parts of the lung tissue become solidified and airless. The general character and extent of the pneumonia lesions or injuries to the tissue, depend largely on the cause and the particular type of pneumonia in individual cases.

Pneumonia may be caused by specific infections, by certain environmental conditions, such as chilling due to exposure, which reduces the defensive forces of the body against disease or by the presence of parasites. Pneumonia caused by parasitism, however, is very rare in cattle. The presence of foreign material in the lungs also may cause what is called mechanical pneumonia; this may, for example, follow treatment by drenching for some other disease.

In any one of its various forms, pneumonia usually progresses through several stages, terminating either in recovery or in the death of the animal.

As a primary disease, pneumonia usually follows chilling caused by exposure to cold winds and rain or to cold, damp quarters. Calves readily contract the disease when exposed directly to drafts when indoors. Overcrowding of young animals in quarters where the air becomes foul, followed by exposure to outside conditions, is also thought to cause pneumonia. When pneumonia is caused by specific types of infection, it is generally a secondary condition accompanying some other disease. It occurs as one of the symptoms of a number of specific diseases of cattle.

Pneumonia is usually characterized in the beginning by dullness, lack of appetite, high temperature, which may reach 107° F, rapid and shallow respiration and dilated nostrils. The pulse is strong and hard, becoming more rapid as the disease progresses. A cough mayor may not be present in the early stages. The muzzle is hot and dry. The coat is usually rough and the skin rather dry. Constipation may or may not be present, but usually, as the disease progresses, diarrhoea occurs. The animal assumes positions that facilitate easier breathing. It may stand with the forefeet spread apart, for example or rest on the sternum when lying down.

On close examination, sounds may be heard over the chest wall, varying from a slight wheezing noise to a gurgling or splashing sounds depending on the stage to which the disease has developed and also on the amount of lung tissue involved. A discharge from the nostrils may be present, varying from a small quantity of clear fluid to a large amount of sticky, pale yellow material. The course of the disease is variable. Death may follow within a few days after the onset of symptoms, recovery may occur in an equally short time or the disease may become chronic and persist for several weeks.

In the diagnosis of pneumonia, a history of drenching for some other condition would be strongly indicative of the mechanical type. When only one animal in a herd is affected and there is no suspicion of a contagious or infectious disease, the primary type of pneumonia, as from exposure, would be suspected.

In the treatment of pneumonia, good hygienic surroundings, protection from drafts, wind and rain and other provisions for the comfort of the animal are essential. When the animal is on the road to recovery, palatable, easily digested foods in small amounts should be given frequently. Medicinal treatment consists in giving various tonis and stimulants. The application of counter irritants, such as mustard plasters, is practiced by many. No specific treatment in the form of sera and vaccines, as in the case of human pneumonia, has been developed, though the administration of specific antisera may be beneficial if the pneumonia is secondary to some specific infectious disease for which the specific antiserum is available. There are reports of very beneficial results in pneumonic conditions from the use of large injections of blood from normal cattle. In recent years considerable experimental work has been done in the treatment of pneumonia with the sulfonamide drugs. Although some encouraging results have been reported, further studies must be carried out before specific recommendations regarding the use of these drugs can be made.

Since pneumonia is encountered in so many forms and stages, the proper treatment of the disease is a problem for the trained veterinarian.

Choke

Choke in cattle is caused by an attempt to swallow large objects without thoroughly chewing them. Swallowing food without completely chewing it is characteristic of cattle. Such food materials as ears of corn, beets, apples, turnips, pieces of cabbage or cabbage stumps and potatoes, are the principal causes of choke. Foreign bodies, such as balls, pieces o metal, glass and even table forks, have been found to be responsible for choke. Some animals, however, may have certain defects or alterations of the normal structure of the esophagus or gullet, such as a narrowing or constriction at some point and when such an animal is hungry and eats greedily, even soft foods like meal, bran or pulp may become lodged in the esophagus and cause choke.

The object swallowed that causes choke may be located either in the neck or in the chest portion of the esophagus and it may or may not be large enough to completely obstruct the passages of water to the stomach and air to the lungs. The symptoms and the gravity of the condition depend largely on the character, size and location of the obstruction. Generally, the first symptoms observed are restlessness, salivation, retching, forced swallowing movements and coughing. The animal will not attempt to eat or drink, particularly if the obstruction is lodged in the part of the gullet in the region of the neck. Bloating will occur eventually, adding to the discomfort of the animal. If the offending object is located In the chest portion of the esophagus or if it is small enough in size to allow passage of gas and air, the early symptoms may not be particularly alarming and the animal may even try to eat or drink. The food is promptly regurgitated and coughing and retching follow.

Treatment to remove the obstruction will depend on its location, size and character. If the object is an article of food lodged in the neck portion of the esophagus, it should be forced upward as gently as possible to the pharynx, at the back of the mouth cavity, by placing a hand on either side of the neck, along the jugular furrow and pressing upward against the object. When it reaches the pharynx it can be removed by the hand through the animal's mouth.

If the object is in the chest portion of the esophagus, its removal will require a different procedure. The use of a stomach tube with a slender rod called a probang inserted at the end has proved quite efficient for this purpose. The tube, which is flexible and one-half to 1 inch in diameter, with an aperture for the insertion of the wooden probang, will follow the natural curvature of the neck. It should first be lubricated with linseed oil or some other harmless oil, then carefully inserted through the mouth into the esophagus and gently pushed downward until the obstruction is encountered. Firm but gentle continuous pressure is then applied. If it is impossible to push the object on into the rumen or first stomach, by this method operative procedure, requiring the services of a veterinarian, may be necessary.

A doubled-wire loop, sufficiently heavy or stiff to allow manipulation, is frequently used by veterinarians in removing foreign objects from the esophagus of cattle, regardless of the location.

Rough procedures, such as pushing too hard with the tube and probang or trying to crush an object such as an apple or beet between blocks of wood or bricks, are to be avoided, since there is danger of causing serious injury to the tissues of the throat that may result in the death of the animal. When there is bloating or distension of the rumen with gas, it may be necessary to alleviate this condition before attempting to remove the obstruction from the esophagus. Sometimes it is possible to pass the tube with the probang inserted past the object and into the rumen. The probang is then withdrawn, permitting quantities of gas to escape and relieving the condition. In other cases it may be necessary to insert a trochar or surgical probe, through the abdominal wall in order to bring about relief.

The symptoms of choke in most cases are quite alarming, but sudden death seldom occurs. The object may sometimes become dislodged in 1 to 2 days without mechanical assistance of any kind. During this time, of course, bloat develops and must necessarily be relieved occasionally. In the case of a valuable animal, the assistance of a veterinarian should be obtained promptly.

Literature Cited

(1) BARDENS, G.W. (1938). TREATMENT OF INFECTIOUS KERATITIS WITH MERCUROCHROME. Amer. Vet. Med. Assoc. Jour. 93: 35-36.

(2) BENGSTON. JOHN S. (1938). PRIMARY RETICULUM CELL SARCOMA OF THE LYMPH NODES OF A COW WITH WIDESPRED METASTASES. Amer. Jour. Path. 14: 365-376.

(3) CREECH, G.T. (1935). PRIMARY ACTINOMYCOSIS OF THE PERITONEUM OF YOUNG CALVES. Bull. Vet. 11 (4): [1]-2, illus.

(4) CREECH, G.T. and BUNYEA, HUBERT (1929). EXPERIMENTAL STUDIES OF BOVINE LEUKEMIA. Jour. Agr. Res. 38: 395-404, illus.

(5) _______and MILLER, F.W. (1933). NASAL GRANULOMA IN CATTLE. Vet. Med. 28: 279-284, illus.

(6) DIKMANS, G. (1934). NASAL GRANULOMA IN CATTLE IN LOUISIANA. North Amer. Vet. 15 (9): 20-24, illus.

(7) FELDMAN, WILLIAM HUGH (1932). NEOPLASMS OF DOMESTICATED ANIMALS. 410 pp, illus., Philadelphia and London.

(8) KALKUS, J.W. (1920). A STUDY OF GOITRE AND ASSOCIATED CONDITIONS IN DOMESTIC ANIMALS. Wash. Agr. Expt. Sta. Bul. 156, 48 pp, illus.

(9) KANSAS AGKIOULTURAL EXPERIMENTSTATION (1938). FEEDER CATTLE INVESTIGATIONS. Kans. Agr. Expt. Sta. Bien. Rpt. (1936-38) 9: 113-114.

(10) MOBRILL, C. C. & GRAHAM, ROBERT (1941). AN OUTBREAK OF BOVINE PSEUDORABIES OR MAD ITCH. Amer. Jour. Vet. Res. 2 (2): 35-40, illus.

(11) MURRAY, CHAS (1933). MAD ITCH. Cornell Vet. 23: 303-305, illus.

(12) ROSSING, T.E. (1936). A CASE OF PSEUDO RABIES OR (MAD ITCH). Fort Dodge Bio-chemic Rev. 7(3): 20-21, illus.

(13) SHOPE, RIOHARD E. (1931). AN EXPERIMENTAL STUDY OF "MAD ITCH," WITH ESPECIAL REFERENCE TO ITS RELATIONSHIP TO PSEUDORABIES. Jour. Expt. Med. 54: 233-248.

Chapter 8

CATTLE COCCIDIOSIS

Donald C. Boughton[1]

[1] Donald C. Boughton is Associate Protozoologist, Regional Animal Disease Research Laboratory, Auburn, Ala., Bureau of Animal Industry.

An infectious intestinal disease caused by a minute parasite, coccidiosis sometimes causes heavy losses among calves. An uninfected calf is the exception rather than the rule, because carriers of the disease are everywhere. There is no cure, but careful management and sanitation can go along way toward prevention.

Bovine coccidiosis is an infectious disease of cattle, known in its spectacular form as bloody scours or red diarrhoea because of the characteristic bloody fecal discharges seen in severe cases. The disease is of economic importance in many parts of the world, including the United States (*1, 12, 15*).[2] To the outright loss from fatal infections, which may take a heavy toll among calves, must be added the no less significant loss from retarded growth and general unthriftiness among survivors of nonfatal infections, many of which go undiagnosed because marked clinical symptoms are lacking.

Nature of the Disease

Coccidiosis is essentially intestinal malaria. The microscopic, one-celled animal parasites, called coccidia, that cause it are close relatives of malaria organisms. As in malaria, a knowledge of the

[2] Italic numbers in parentheses refer to Literature Cited.

two-phase life cycle of the parasites is of fundamental importance. Whereas the malaria parasites utilize the blood cells, the coccidia invade the intestinal lining of their victim. The injury to the host occurs during this phase of the coccidian life cycle. After a period of multiplication within the intestinal tissues, coccidia produce resistant forms, known as oocysts, which are discharged in the feces. Outside the animal they live a nonparasitic existence until picked up by a new victim. This second phase is obviously responsible for the transmission of the disease. Malaria parasites, on the other hand, are trapped in the blood stream and require the aid of a mosquito to make the transfer from one host to another.

A significant feature of bovine coccidiosis is that the massive multiplication of the parasites within the host does not continue indefinitely but is culminated rather abruptly with the discharge of large numbers of oocysts. Following natural exposure or experimental inoculation, the oocysts appear in the dung in from 1 to 3 weeks, depending on the species of coccidia involved. Reproduction of the parasites appears to be self-limited (*14*). Possibly the length of the multiplication period may be affected by host reaction (*15*). In any event, at least two points of practical significance depend upon this limitation on multiplication. In the first place, infection is often of short duration and recovery consequently spontaneous. Claims for successful treatment must be judged in the light of this fact. Second, the final number of coccidia within the host's tissues at the end of the multiplication period is likely to be smaller if only a few infective oocysts were ingested. Other things being equal, small numbers of coccidia produce less damage than large numbers. The severity of an infection, therefore, depends on the number of parasites introduced into the intestinal lining.

Acute outbreaks of bovine coccidiosis often appear where young animals are crowded together. This is in line with the general observation that coccidiosis becomes of economic importance wherever mass production of animals involves crowding of the host population (*14*). Groups of calves confined in small lots are more often heavily infected than calves on pasture. Acute infections may appear among yearlings confined in feed lots at the end of the grazing season. Two factors are generally held to be responsible for outbreaks when young or previously unexposed older animals are confined in close quarters:

(1) Such animals have less resistance than those that have already experienced infection, and

(2) They are exposed to a relatively high concentration of parasites.

Injuries Produced and Symptoms

The injuries produced by coccidiosis in cattle result directly or indirectly from massive multiplication (asexual reproduction) of coccidia within the linings of the small intestine, cecum, colon or rectum. Resulting gross lesions include:

(1) Loss of surface epithelium or lining membrane;

(2) Thickening of the mucous membrane, with the formation of irregular, whitish ridges; and

(3) Hemorrhages, which may be petechial–of pinpoint size–in mild cases and diffuse in acute cases. Catarrhal enteritis (intestinal inflammation) is often present in both the small and the large intestines.

Symptoms associated with this condition are bloody diarrhoea, anemia, weakness and general emaciation. Severe straining accompanies the voiding of feces, which may consist primarily of stringy masses of mucus and blood. Secondary bacterial infection-another disease coming on top of the first one–is a common sequel. Pneumonia often develops. An animal that does not die within a week or two after the onset of an acute attack may be expected to recover rather promptly from the diarrhoea and improve gradually in general condition.

Calves, often during the second month of life, may suffer from rather severe but nonfatal coccidial infections which fail to produce marked symptoms. There is a more or less persistence nonbloody diarrhoea, which has often been mistaken for a prolongation of white scours. Affected animals are unthrifty and often fail to make normal gains in weight.

Transmission

The ultimate source of the parasites causing bovine coccidiosis is an infected bovine host. Formerly it was thought that all coccidia found in the various domestic and wild animals belonged to the same species. Sparrows, for example, were accused (*8*), falsely, as it was shown later (*4*), of harboring poultry coccidia. Cross-infection experiments, however, have proved that with a few exceptions the different coccidia are specific to their own hosts. None of the species of cattle coccidia tested have been found to infect other animals, such as rabbits, sheep, goats, swine, guinea pigs, rats, mice and chickens (*7, 16, 18*). Coccidial infections of nonbovine origin have not been demonstrated in cattle, which are undoubtedly exposed while grazing to coccidia of various invertebrate, avian and mammalian hosts.

Coccidial infection in cattle that do not show clinical symptoms is common. Surveys of wild and domesticated animals have revealed high percentages of infected individuals (*2, 3, 9, 10, 11, 12*). As a matter of fact, an uninfected calf is the exception rather than the rule. Although special concentration techniques may be required to discover the coccidia, they can often be found in healthy adult cattle and the actual number of oocysts discharged during a given period, say a month, is enormous. Such healthy animals harboring the organisms are known as carriers of coccidiosis. The carrier state probably involves repeated infection and, possibly to a limited extent, the prolongation of low-grade parasite reproduction following an attack. Second and subsequent infections, under ordinary management practices, are usually milder than first infections, presumably because resistance is increased and exposure is reduced. Carriers are a constant source of oocysts.

Bovine coccidiosis is transmitted by means of the infective oocysts, which, as already pointed out, must be of bovine origin. Following the parasitic phase within the host, undeveloped oocysts are discharged in the feces. Large numbers are characteristic of severe, nonfatal infections; small numbers may be discharged by carriers, presumably as the result of mild reinfection with the same species or new infections with different species. The majority of the oocysts from a single infection may often be eliminated in the short period of 3 to 6 days.

Before an oocyst becomes infective, the living material within the cyst wall must undergo a development (sporulation) which requires 2 to 6 days under the most favorable conditions of oxygen and moisture (*3, 15, 16*). This is a vulnerable period in the coccidian life cycle during which sanitary measures can operate successfully. If manure were removed daily, the freshly passed oocysts would not have time to become infective. Oocysts are resistant and can remain alive for several months in fecal material in a barn or pasture. Large numbers are often plastered on the coat of a calf befouled with manure, where they are readily accessible to the calf's tongue. Oocysts can be destroyed by drying and by strong disinfectants. Strong solutions of lye or bichloride of mercury are effective when applied to walls and floors by means of a stiff brush. When an infective oocyst is ingested by a susceptible calf, the cyst wall is digested, releasing eight small forms (sporozoites) within. The latter penetrate the cells of the lining membrane of the digestive tract, where they begin parasitic multiplication.

Species of Coccidia Involved

There are at least 10 species of bovine coccidia (*3, 13*). This fact complicates and at the same time helps to clarify studies on bovine coccidiosis; generalizations regarding the disease must be qualified and conflicting observations interpreted on the basis of the individual species involved. It is believed that all the species belong to the genus *Eimeria*, the report of a bovine *Isospora* (*5*) not having been verified. At present, species differentiation is based on the following' traits:

(1) Characteristics of the oocyst, such as size, shape, color, micropyle, residual body;

(2) Structure of sporocysts;

(3) Sporulation time;

(4) Specific immunities developed; and

(5) Length of time between inoculation and appearance of oocysts.

The following species are recognized at present: *E. alabanmensis, E. auburnensis, E. bovis, E. brasiliensis, E. bukidnonesis, E. canodensis, E. cylindrica, E. ellipsoidalis, E. subspherica, E. zurnii.* Description of tissue stages and the relative pathological significance of individual species await further investigation. There is evidence, however, which indicates that certain species, notably *E. zurnii, E. ellipsoidalis* and *E. bovis*, are of greater economic importance than the others (*1, 3, 15* and unpublished data).

Control and Treatment

Control of coccidial infection and prevention of clinical coccidiosis are based upon two fundamental facts: (1) coccidiosis carriers are universally present and (2) excessive exposure to coccidia is particularly harmful to young stock. Sanitary measures and management practices must be designed to prevent young calves from ingesting large numbers of infective oocysts.

A very common serious mistake is to introduce young calves directly into a group of calves of various ages confined in close quarters. Such conditions are ideal for producing severe infections, as the following typical chain of events indicates: Since coccidia, distributed by carriers, are universally present, the first few calves in a given lot are bound to pick up a few stray oocysts. As a result, these calves develop nonclinical infections and discharge large numbers of oocysts. Calves subsequently added to the group are exposed to increasingly large numbers of oocysts and their infections and discharges, in turn, raise the parasite population to a dangerous level.

Isolation of young dairy calves, as in individual box stalls, does much to prevent heavy infections. Daily removal of manure and wet, contaminated bedding is important. Precautions must be taken to avoid the introduction of fecal material from other places by the shoes of the caretaker, for example, at feeding time. The use of individual milk pails, cleaned thoroughly between feedings, is advantageous. Calves up to 6, weeks of age should not be removed from their stalls, even during the short period required for cleaning, unless special care is taken to prevent contact with other cattle and unsterilized objects.

Where isolation of dairy calves is impractical and the quarters are not cleaned daily, segregation of calves by ages is helpful. For example, separate pens for different age groups may be provided as follows:

(1) For calves under 3 weeks old,

(2) For calves 3 to 6 weeks old,

(3) For calves 6 weeks to 3 months old, and

(4) For calves over 3 months old.

The two youngest groups require particular attention. The upper age limit of the third group is chosen more for convenience in caring for the animals than for any practical advantage in reducing coccidial infection.

The first pen, shed or lot, assigned to the youngest group, is used exclusively for these animals, calves of all other ages being excluded at all times. Upon reaching the 3-week age limit, all calves are removed promptly from the first pen and placed in the second pen. Because oocysts are rarely discharged by calves under 3 weeks of age, the first pen can be kept free from large numbers of oocysts. Newborn calves subsequently introduced are spared severe infections, which have serious consequences in very young animals and are given an opportunity to gain in bodily vigor and to begin normal growth before being exposed to the older animals in the second pen. Nonclinical infections may be expected to develop in the first few calves introduced into the second pen; the short stay here is designed to prevent the excessive accumulation of infective oocysts which might otherwise take place as the calves subsequently introduced become infected.

It goes without saying that sanitary measures are not to be abandoned upon the adoption of some such age-segregation plan. It is profitable to go to some pains to protect calves against severe coccidiosis in the early weeks of life, inasmuch as thereafter they are usually able to withstand the coccidial infections to which they will almost certainly be subjected.

Where large herds of beef or dairy stock are fed outdoors, the wet, muddy ground around haystacks, feed sheds and watering troughs presents a special problem. Low spots should be filled in and proper drainage provide so as to permit the ground to dry out from time to time. Manure should be picked up daily if practicable. If contamination proves to be excessive, a change of feeding place is indicated.

Treatment is entirely for the relief of symptoms and include the judicious administration of astringents and intestinal antiseptics. and measures designed to prevent reinfection and maintain bodily vigor. A specific drug for bovine coccidiosis is not known. The beneficial results claimed for various types of drug treatments that have been employed from time to time (*6, 17*) may often be due in reality to spontaneous cure under favorable hygienic conditions.

Recent experiments made by the writer with sulfaguanidine, however, suggest that this drug holds promise for the future.

Literature Cited

(1) BECKER, ELERY R. (1934). COCCIDIA AND COCCIDIOSIS OF DOMESTICATED, GAME AND LABORATORY ANIMALS AND OF MAN. 147 pp, illus. Ames, Iowa. (Iowa State Col., Div. of Indus. Sci., Monog. 2.)

(2) BOUGHTON, DONALD C. (1937). NOTES ON AVIAN COCCIDIOSIS. Auk 54: 500-509, illus.

(3) CHRISTENSEN, JOHN F. (1941). THE OOCYSTS OF COCCIDIA FROM DOMESTIC CATTLE IN ALABAMA (U.S.A.), WITH DESCRIPTIONS OF TWO NEW SPECIES. Jour. Parasitol. 27: 203-220, illus.

(4) CLELAND, J.B. (1914). INTESTINAL COCCIDIOSIS IN HOUSE SPARROWS (PASSER DOMESTICUS) IN NEW SOUTH WALES. *In* 3d Rpt. Govt. Bur. of Microbiol., New South Wales (1912), p. 134.

(5) COOPER, HUGH, & GULATI, AMARNATH (1926). ON THE OCCURRENCE OF ISOSPORA AND BALANTIDIUM IN CATTLE. India Dept. Agr. Mem., Vet. Ser., 3: 191-193, illus.

(6) FRANK, E.R. (1926). COCCIDIOSIS IN FEEDER CATTLE. Amer. Vet. Med. Assoc. Jour. 69: 729-733.

(7) GUILLEBEAU, A. (1893). UEBER DAS VORKOMMEN VON COCCIDIUM OVIFORME BEI DER ROTEN RUHR DES RINDES. (Referat) Zentbl. f. Bakt. [etc.] Originale (I) 14: 467-468.

(8) HADLEY, PHILIP B. (1910). STUDIES IN AVIAN COCCIDIOSIS. III. COCCIDIOSIS IN THE ENGLISH SPARROW AND OTHER WILD BIRDS. Zentbl. f. Bakt. [etc] Originale (I) 56: 522-523.

(9) MARSH, HADLEIGH (1938). HEALTHY CATTLE AS CARRIERS OF COCCIDIA. Amer. Vet. Med. Assoc. Jour. (n.s. 45) 92 (2): 184-194, illus.

(10) ROBERTSON, ANDREW (1931). COCCIDIOSIS IN CALVES. Vet. Jour. 87: 312-325; 351-385, illus.

(11) SKIDMORE, LOUIS V. (1933). BOVINE COCCIDIA CARRIERS. (Abstract) Jour. Parasitol. 20: 126.

(12) SMITH, THEOBALD and GRAYBILL, H.W. (1918). COCCIDIOSIS IN YOUNG CALVES. Jour. Expt. Med. 28: 89-108, illus.

(13) TORRES, SILVIO and RAMOS, J. ILDEFONSO (1939) EIMERIAS DOS BOVINOS EM PERNAMBUCO. Arquivos do Inst. de Pesquisas Agronomicas 2: [79]-96, illus.

(14) TYZZER, ERNEST EDWARD (1929). COCCIDIOSIS IN GALLINACEOUS BIRDS. Amer. Jour. Hyg. 10: 269-383, illus.

(15) WILSON, IRE DONAKER (1931). STUDY OF BOVINE COCCIDIOSIS. Va. Agr. Expt. Sta., Tech. Bul. 42, 42 pp., illus.

(16) WILSON, IRE DONAKER and MORLEY, L.C. (1933). STUDY OF BOVINE COCCIDIOSIS. Amer. Vet. Med. Assoc. Jour. 82: 826-850.

(17) YAKIMOFF, W.L. (1927). LE TRAITEMENT DE LA COCCIDIOSE DES BOVIDES PAR L'ICHTHARGAN. Soc. de Path. Exot. Bul. 20: 588-589.

(18) _______and GALOUZO, J.G. (1927). ZUR FRAGE UBER RINDERCOCCIDIEN. Arch. f. Protistenk. 58: 185-200, illus.

Chapter 9

CATTLE TICK FEVER

W.M. Mac Kellar[1]

[1] *W.M. MacKellar is Principal Veterinarian and Chief. Division of Tick Eradication and Special Diseases, Bureau of Animal Industry.*

The fight to eliminate the cattle fever tick from the United States is probably the most extensive and sustained campaign ever made on any of man's parasitic enemies. Today 99 percent of the formerly infested area has been freed; the once appalling losses have been practically eliminated.

In 1906 a concerted effort to eradicate the cattle fever tick from the United States was begun. At that time and for more than a century before, this infectious disease of cattle and the parasite that transmits it were the most serious obstacles faced by the cattle industry in 15 Southern and Southwestern States the combined area of which constitutes nearly one-fourth of the United States. Conservative estimates in the early 1900's placed the losses directly and indirectly chargeable to this plague at $ 40,000,000 annually.

At different times and places the disease has been known by many different names. The one by which it has been best known in the United States is "Texas fever," but this name is misleading because it gives the wholly erroneous impression that the disease originated in Texas or that it is confined to that State. It has also been known as red water, black water, southern cattle fever, acclimation fever, murrain, bloody murrain, Mexican fever, Spanish fever, splenic or splenetic fever, hemaglobinuria, bovine piroplasmosis and bovine malaria. Since in natural infection the disease is transmitted by one means only, the bite of the cattle fever tick (*Boophilus annulatus*), "cattle tick fever" would seem to describe it best and this is the name now in general use in the United States.

Symptoms

Cattle tick fever is a specific infectious disease of the blood of cattle, caused by the development and activity of minute animal parasites known as piroplasms, which are conveyed to the animals by the cattle fever tick. The disease is characterized by high fever, destruction of red corpuscles, enlarged spleen, engorged liver, thick flaky bile, more or less jaundice, emaciation and death in 10 percent of the chronic to 90 per cent of the acute cases. A peculiarity of the disease is that the animals responsible for its spread are apparently healthy, while those that become diseased do not as a rule convey the infection to others.

A Notable Discovery in Medical Science

Just when or where cattle tick fever first made its appearance in the United States is not known. The generally accepted theory is that it was introduced into the West Indies and Mexico during the Spanish colonization of those countries and from there reached the southern part of the United States. What seems to be the earliest report in this country of a disease which was undoubtedly cattle tick fever was made in 1796; in August of that year there was an outbreak of a cattle disease in Lancaster County, Pa., which was attributed to a drove of cattle previously brought from South Carolina. In every instance in which these southern cattle mingled with native cattle the disease was contracted by the latter and in one instance it was supposed to have been caused by merely placing Pennsylvania cattle on ground where the southern cattle had been penned. It was also noted that outbreaks of this strange malady invariably occurred in summer and would disappear with the first heavy frost and that the southern cattle apparently responsible for spreading the disease Seemed to be in perfect health.

About the middle of the nineteenth century similar accounts of this trouble in the West and Southwest began to be heard. This was the period of the great trail movement of cattle from Texas to the stock-raising sections of the West and because of the enormous losses that followed in the wake of these overland movements the name of

Texas became linked with the malady. Laws and regulations aimed at controlling these movements and preventing the spread of the disease were enacted by several States, but not with standing these local efforts the borderline of the infected area continued to advance northward. This finally led to the conclusion that the problem was of national interest and that if the cattle industry of the North was to be protected it would be necessary for the Federal Government to establish control measures dividing the infected areas from the free areas and regulating the movement of all cattle from the areas where the disease existed.

With this in view, in 1883 a survey was undertaken in an effort to locate the northern limits of the infection and on July 3, 1889, by order of the, Secretary of Agriculture, the first national quarantine order establishing a Federal quarantine line and controlling the movement of, southern cattle was Issued. This quarantine and the strict enforcement of regulations to permit the shipment of southern cattle to northern markets for immediate slaughter only and under special quarantine restrictions proved quite effective in checking the spread of the disease but did little to improve conditions in the quarantine area.

During this time many scientists were conducting investigations in an effort to solve the baffling problems presented by the disease and in 1889 investigators of the Bureau of Animal Industry had the distinction of being the first to recognize and describe as protozoa the intracellular parasites that are the direct causative agents.

Some observing cattlemen of the West had for a long time advanced the theory that Texas fever was caused by ticks, which were carried to and scattered on the northern pastures by southern cattle. Others ridiculed this theory. The Bureau of Animal Industry decided to investigate it and the conclusive experiments conducted by its scientists Dr. Theobald Smith and Dr. Fred L. Kilborne in 1889 and 1890 established the fact that cattle tick infestation was necessary in the transmission of the disease. They thus showed irrefutably and for the first time that an infectious disease could be transmitted by an intermediate host or carrier from one animal to another. About that time Dr. Cooper Curtice, also of the Bureau of Animal Industry, made note-worthy contributions to knowledge of this subject by his studies and description of the life history of the cattle tick. This pioneer work opened a new field in medical science and pointed the way for studies that later solved the problems of the spread of such diseases as malaria, yellow fever, Rocky Mountain spotted fever, typhus and others.

The Tick-Eradication Campaign

There are in the United States two varieties of the cattle fever tick which are responsible for the spread of tick fever–the North American fever tick (*Boophilus annulatus*), which formerly infested most of the quarantined area and the tropical variety of the same tick, *Boophilus annulatus* var. *microplus*, found in Florida, Puerto Rico and areas adjacent to the Gulf coast. This tropical variety has frequently been taken from deer and its ability to perpetuate itself on these wild animals has greatly complicated the eradication problem and delayed completion of tick eradication in some of the large swampy areas of Florida.

Without the tick the disease is of little importance and would probably die out. Recognition of this fact naturally led to investigation as to the feasibility of tick eradication and this resulted in 1906 in the inauguration of a campaign to eliminate cattle ticks from the United States. This work, in which State officials, livestock owners and the Bureau of Animal Industry have cooperated, has continued to the present time. When the cooperative project was undertaken, 985 counties in 15 Southern and Southwestern States were under Federal quarantine because of tick infestation. By December 15, 1940, the tick-eradication campaign had reduced this area to 2 quarantined counties in Florida, where the presence of tick-infested deer has delayed completion of the work and to parts of 8 counties adjacent to the Rio Grande in Texas, where infestation continues to filter in on stray and smuggled animals from Mexico.

Medicinal treatment of cattle sick with tick fever had usually been unsatisfactory and it was generally believed in the United States that the disease and other losses chargeable to the tick could be satisfactorily and finally disposed of only by its complete elimination. Official work since 1906 has had that end in view. It was sometimes desirable, however, to ship well-bred cattle to infected districts in the South or to export them to tick-infested countries. These cattle, therefore, were immunized so that they could be introduced into the infected areas with comparatively little loss from the fever. Immunity was obtained by introducing the microparasite into the system by blood inoculation. It was found that young animals 6 to 15 months old best withstood this treatment and were more readily and completely immunized than older animals.

The eradication of the fever ticks is accomplished by killing them on the pastures and on the cattle. Pastures may be rendered tick-free by excluding all the host animals–cattle, horses and mules–until all the ticks on the ground have died of starvation. The other and more common method is to let the cattle remain on the infested pastures and disinfect the animals at regular intervals, usually every 2 weeks, by dipping in an arsenical solution. This prevents the engorged female ticks from dropping to the ground alive and reinfesting the pastures. The seed ticks that are on the ground and those that hatch from eggs laid by females already there will get on the cattle from time to time and be destroyed by the dipping, while those that fail to find a host will starve to death. The length of time it will be necessary to continue the systematic dipping to insure eradication varies somewhat with the time of year the dipping starts and with the thoroughness of the work. The most satisfactory results have followed when dipping began in March and was continued at 14-day intervals until November.

Losses Due Directly to Cattle Ticks

The cattle fever tick is of great importance as the only natural agent by which cattle tick fever is transmitted from animal to animal and eradication of the tick will result in eliminating the disease. But even if this were not the case, the damage done by the tick as an external parasite would more than justify the trouble and expense of the eradication effort.

The only food of the cattle fever tick is blood and the loss of the blood it takes from cattle in its rapid development impoverishes the animals (Fig. 1). Heavy infestation means that cattle must have more feed merely to meet the demands of the parasites; the growth of young animals is retarded and they may remain thin, weak; and stunted (Fig. 2A). In dairy cows, the milk flow is greatly reduced.

Since May 1, 1928, the interstate shipment of tick-infested cattle for any purpose has been prohibited. This has necessitated the trouble and expense of dipping the cattle and freeing then of ticks before shipment. Formerly cattle coming from an infested district and sold in the "southern pens" at northern markets brought from

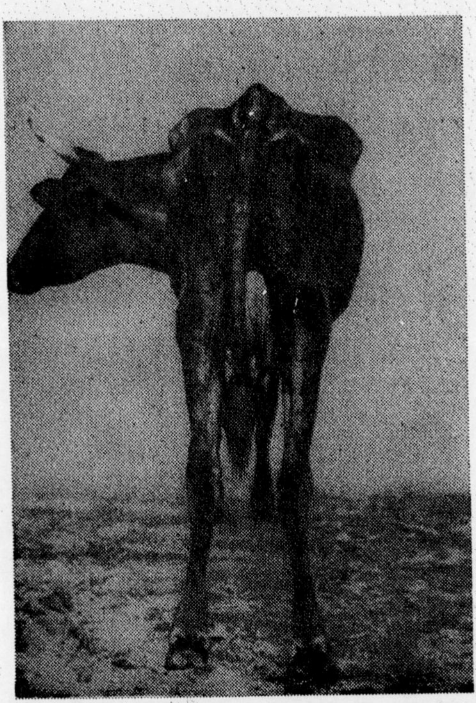

Fig. 1: A cow emaciated by heavy infestation with the cattle fever tick. This condition was once common in cattle throughout the South, but it is no longer seen in the United States.

1½ to 1½ cents a pound less than the quoted market prices. The cars used in shipping southern cattle had to be cleaned and disinfected, which added to the cost of transportation. The handicap placed on cattle raisers as a result of the decreased value of their stock averaged, at the figure quoted, from $3 to $9 a head, allowing an average weight of 600 pounds for all classes of cattle. This decreased value was reflected in the valuation of all cattle in the quarantined area and the value of the infested ranges and pastures was also lowered, reducing the assets of the whole section. Tick infestation not only

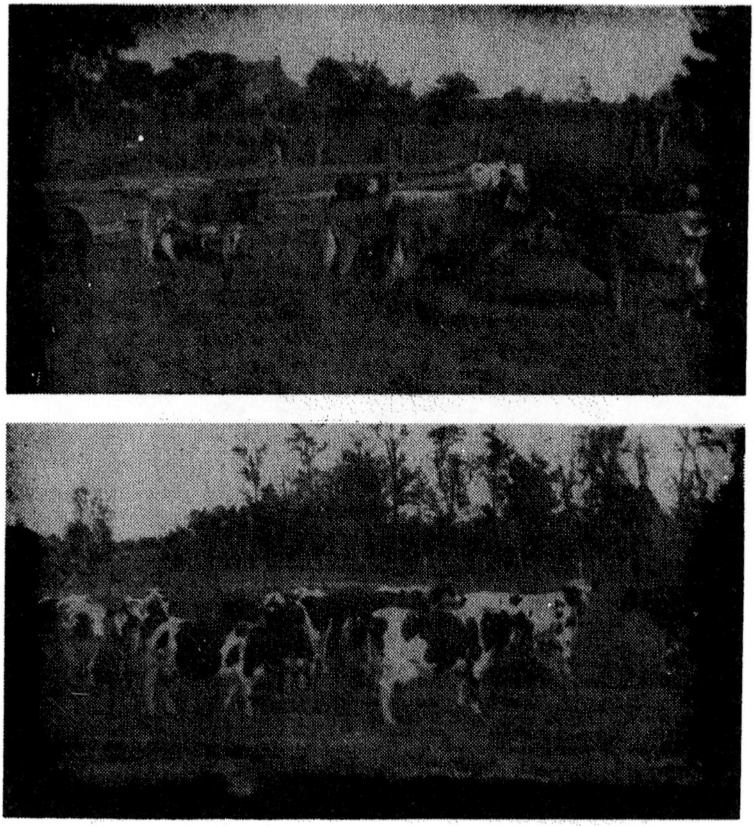

Fig. 2*A*: A typical herd of ticky cattle; *B*: Improved cattle in an area freed of ticks.

lessened the value of the live animals but caused their hides to be graded as of No. 4 quality. The same hide if free from ticks would grade No. 2 and the difference in price between these two grades is 3 to 5 cents a pound. Since a steer hide weighs about 42 pounds, the presence of ticks caused a loss in the hide alone of $1.25 to $2.10. The losses sustained by southern purchasers of northern purebred cattle with which to improve the native stock was another important item. About 10 percent of such cattle, even if immunized, would die of cattle tick fever and 60 percent or more would succumb if they were not so treated

The Greatest of All Campaigns Against Parasites

The fight to eliminate the cattle fever tick from the United States is probably the most extensive and sustained attack ever made on any of man's parasitic enemies. It has resulted in freeing approximately 99 percent of the area formerly infested and has almost entirely eliminated the appalling losses once caused by the tick in the beef and dairy industries of the South. Death losses from tick fever have been practically eliminated. The last report of an outbreak of the disease was in August 1939. Special pens for southern cattle at northern market centers are a thing of the past; southern cattle now move to market or elsewhere without restrictions and compete on an equal basis with stock from other parts of the country (Fig. 2, B). Purebred breeding animals for the improvement of native cattle may now be shipped to any part of the South without fear of loss from tick fever and this has resulted in a marked improvement in recent years in the quality of southern cattle. The total cost to the cooperating State, county and Federal Governments of eliminating this pest will amount to little more than the toll taken from the South in a single year by the cattle fever tick before eradication was undertaken.

Chapter 10

ANAPLASMOSIS: A DISEASE OF CATTLE

George W. Stiles[1]

[1] *George W. Stiles is Bacteriologist in Charge, Branch Pathological Laboratory, Denver, Colo., Bureau of Animal Industry.*

Anaplasmosis is a serious blood disease of cattle and it is slowly spreading to new areas. Much has been found out about the ways in which it is transmitted, but a preventive or a cure is still to be discovered by research.

Anaplasmosis was probably introduced into the United States by the Spaniards at the same time that splenic or cattle tick fever entered this country (*13*).[2] The disease, which is not transmissible to man, chiefly affects cattle, although the antelope, black wildebeest, blesbok, buffalo, camel, deer, duiker, elk, goat and sheep are reported to be susceptible.

Mature cattle are more subject to infection than young animals. Although calves doubtless acquire mild cases, they are seldom observed to be sick or dying in anaplasmosis-infected herds. Cattle of all breeds may acquire the disease. Some immunity appears to develop in herds in which anaplasmosis has long been prevalent, but a few authentic cases have been reported of a second attack after a year in cows that have recovered.

---

[2] Italic numbers In parentheses refer to Literature Cited.

Anaplasmosis is generally considered to be a tropical or semitropical disease, but it also occurs in localities that have low winter temperatures. It has been reported from Africa, Argentina, Brazil and several other South American countries, Cochin-China, France, Italy, Java, the Philippine Islands, the Union of Soviet Socialist Republics and the Island of Taiwan.

In the United States the malady is known to exist in 23 States–Alabama, Arizona, Arkansas, California, Colorado, Delaware, Florida, Georgia, Idaho, Kansas, Louisiana, Maryland, Mississippi, Missouri, Montana, Nevada, North Carolina, Ohio, Oklahoma, Oregon, Texas, Virginia, and Wyoming. It may be present but unrecognized in other States. It is slowly spreading to new areas.

The incidence of anaplasmosis seems to be influenced by climatic conditions favorable to insects and ticks that carry the infection. In the United States natural outbreaks usually occur during the summer and fall. Occasionally cases develop in winter in the South. On the Pacific coast the infection, carried by ticks, is common in winter and spring. The disease occurs more frequently in timbered or brushy wet areas than on dry treeless plains, where most species of ticks, horseflies and mosquitoes are less abundant. Excessive rainfall, floods, irrigation ditches and marshes provide favorable conditions for the propagation of insects and hence opportunities for the transmission of the disease.

Nature and Symptoms of the Disease

Anaplasmosis is an infectious disease caused by a minute parasite which invades the red blood cells and destroys a large number of them, so that the blood becomes pale and watery. Under natural conditions the microparasite is carried from infected to healthy animals by ticks, horseflies, mosquitoes and probably other biting insects, as well as by unclean surgical procedures. (An account of the results of research on the transmission of the disease is given at the end of this article).

In 1910 Theiler (25), of South Africa, described the parasites that cause anaplasmosis as minute, specklike, protozoan bodies in the red cells of the blood and named them *Anaplasma marginale* because of their position near the margin of the cells. Theiler also observed a variety, *A. centrale*, centrally located in the cells and less virulent than the marginal type.[3]

Red blood cells may contain one to three or even more, microparasites (Fig. 1). Early in the course of anaplasmosis only a few of the blood cells contain the parasites, but as the disease progresses the temperature rises, ranging from 103° to 107° F (normal range 100.5° to 102.5°) and the number of red cells involved rapidly increases. Later the temperature drops to normal and may even be subnormal at the time of death. In convalescent cases, the number of parasites lessens, but red cells containing fine granular bodies called stipple cells appear. Cells of this type also occur in other forms of anemia.

In typical cases the heart action is rapid and pounding, with a pulse rate of 70 to 140 a minute (normal range 40 to 70). In severe cases the red-cell blood count usually drops from a normal of about 5 to 1 million per cubic millimeter of blood to 2 million or less. In normal cattle the hemoglobin or blood-color test is approximately 80 (Tallquist scale), whereas in sick animals a color test of 20 to 30 is not uncommon.

In an advanced case the breathing is labored and difficult and the muzzle is dry. There are marked depression, tremors of the muscles, loss of appetite and a great reduction in the milk flow. The skin, teats, udder, vagina, whites of the eyes and all visible membranes become pale and yellow. Pica or depraved appetite, evidenced by the eating of bones or dirt, is not uncommon. Sick animals may show brain symptoms and an inclination to fight.

Dribbling urination is common in anaplasmosis, but the urine is not bloody or wine-colored. Sick cattle are usually constipated and abortion often occurs in advanced pregnancy. Death may follow

---

[3] Some workers claim that the causative agent is a type of filtrable virus notwithstanding the fact that filtered blood from sick animals fails to reproduce the disease Dikmans (*3*) holds that the causative agent may be either a "reaction product," due to a virus, or a "parasite *sui generis*." Du Toit (*4*) says "It is difficult to ascertain why there has been so much reluctance to accept the parasitic theory of anaplasmosis. * * * If we take all the known facts about anaplasmosis into consideration, we come to the conclusion that the simplest and most natural view to take is that this disease is caused by *Anaplasma marginale* and that this organism probably belongs to the Protozoa."

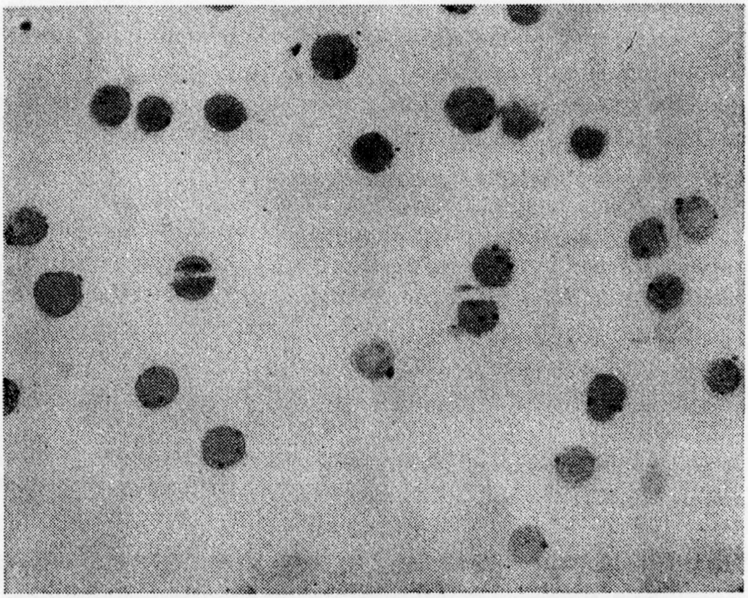

Fig. 1: Red blood cells from a field case of anaplasmosis. The black dots near the margins of the cells are *Anaplasma marginale.* × 1,200.

within 1 or several days after the clinical symptoms of the disease appear. Recovery is usually slow.

There is a wide range in the death rate of affected herds. Sometime from out of a considerable number infected in a herd only one cow may die, but the average death rate usually varies from 25 to 60 percent of the infected animals. When microscopic examination of the blood from a sick cow shows that 40 to 60 percent of the red cells contain marginal bodies, it is probable that the animal will die; if the number of infected red cells is only 10 to 20 percent, it is more likely to recover.

On post mortem examination, cattle dead of anaplasmosis usually show a marked yellow discoloration of the skin, teats and visible mucous membranes. Often the heart is flabby and hemorrhagic blotches may appear on its surface. The blood is thin and watery and the lungs are usually pale and filled with air bubbles.

The liver is enlarged and jaundiced and contents of the bile bladder are dark green, granular and gelatinous in appearance. The spleen or milt, is generally enlarged and soft and in appearance resembles blackberry jam. The urine may be concentrated and slightly darkened. The bowels generally show a catarrhal condition.

Diagnosis

Within quarantine areas anaplasmosis may be mistaken for cattle tick fever. In the latter disease, however, the urine is usually bloody, while in anaplasmosis discolored urine is not the rule. In the Rocky Mountain region the bacterial disease icterohemoglobinuria, described by Vawter and Records (27), may be confused with anaplasmosis; both diseases cause jaundice. In the Midwestern States cattle of all ages are subject to a fairly widespread disease which is characterized by wine-colored urine but about which little else is known. Blood from animals affected with this disease has failed to produce it when injected into healthy cows. Anthrax and hemorrhagic septicemia have been confused with anaplasmosis. A careful bacteriological and microscopic examination and animal inoculations with blood and tissues from infected cattle should definitely determine the diagnosis.

Carrier Animals and Immunization

Unfortunately all cattle that recover from anaplasmosis become carriers. Moreover, it has been shown that the infection may be transmitted from the dam to the unborn calf, which also becomes a carrier. At the Beltsville, Md., station the Bureau of Animal Industry has a cow that is still a proved carrier 13 years after recovery from anaplasmosis. When introduced into clean herds, such animals serve as sources of infection, particularly if ticks or other vectors are present.

In areas where the disease exists only in scattered herds it is prudent to fatten all animals that recover and ship them for slaughter, thus reducing the sources of new infection. In areas where the infection is widespread, involving many herds, the slaughter plan is not altogether practical. The sick animals are treated and those that recover are kept in the herd. The owner should try, however, in every possible way, to prevent the spread of the disease by mechanical or other means.

In some foreign countries, a procedure known as premunition is used to make cattle resistant to anaplasmosis. A small dose of blood from a known carrier is inoculated into the susceptible animal, preferably at an early age (under 6 months) since calves do not react so severely as adult cattle. The vaccinated animals become immune but also become carriers, so that immunization by such vaccination is not recommended in the United States. A number of vaccines prepared by methods designed to destroy the infective agent have been used experimentally, but none have proved successful.

Treatment

The treatment of anaplasmosis is largely a veterinary problem, but the owner can give valuable assistance. Sick animals should be kept in the shade and given plenty of clean water, a little appetizing green feed and protection against flies and mosquitoes. Good nursing is vital. Unnecessary or rough handling of sick cattle, especially range animals, may cause or hasten their death. In drenching cattle with salts, linseed oil or other drugs, care should be taken to prevent the liquid from entering the lungs. Since cattle sick with anaplasmosis are usually constipated, mild saline purges are indicated. Animals that drink a great deal of water freely often recover; therefore, if affected animals do not drink water copiously, large quantities should be given by means of a stomach tube. When weakness develops, veterinarians often use hypodermic injections of camphor or strychnin.

Many drugs are used for the treatment of anaplasmosis. Among these, sodium cacodylate has its advocates, but its value has not been proved by controlled experiments. Injecting carrier cattle with a 10-percent solution of this drug in doses of 30 and 40 grains per 100 pounds of body weight was ineffective in freeing the animals of the microparasites (*26*). A modified sodium cacodylate treatment suggested by Boynton (2) consists in the intravenous injection of 1 liter of 5-percent dextrose in distilled water, to which has been added sufficient sodium cacodylate solution to make a dosage of 25 to 30 grains per 100 pounds of body weight. The cacodylate solution consisted of 4.5 grains of the drug per cubic centimeter of water. The required number of cubic centimeters of this solution was added immediately before injection.

Encouraging results from the intravenous injection of 2- to 4-per cent mercurochrome have been reported by Dykstra and other veterinarians (*5*) .A desirable mild purging action follows the use of this drug.

According to Koger (*10*) large quantities of whole citrated blood from healthy bovines injected intravenously seem to reduce the mortality, especially if given early in the course of the disease. (Citrated blood is blood drawn from a healthy animal into a sodium citrate solution which prevents coagulation and thus facilitates its injection.)

Continued efforts are being made to perfect some specific remedy with which to control and treat anaplasmosis.

Details Concerning the Transmission of Anaplasmosis

Mechanical Spread by Unclean Surgery

During 15 years of field and laboratory experience with anaplasmosis in various parts of the United States, the writer (*23*) has learned of and diagnosed many cases of the disease in herds harboring carriers. The cases followed dehorning or other surgical procedures in which sanitary precautions were not observed.

In temperate climates dehorning and tipping (*6, 12*) are usually done during the cool months to escape screwworm or other fly infestations. Even then, many cases of anaplasmosis have developed following these operations, probably because appropriate precautions were not taken to disinfect instruments between operations.

That contaminated instruments and hypodermic needles can transmit anaplasmosis is supported by experiments by Rees (*16*), who spread the disease by lancet pricks. Sanborn, Stiles and Moe (*20*) reproduced infection by injecting 0.025 cubic centimeter of blood from an acute case intradermically into a healthy cow. Anaplasmosis may be transmitted from carrier animals by unclean needles used in vaccination or in drawing blood, by nose tongs and by castration, slitting of the ears or other surgical procedures.

It is essential that sterile instruments be used for every animal to be bled, injected or operated upon. A sufficient number of bleeding needles should be provided and they should be kept clean and sanitary. Used needles, saws and other instruments should first be washed in cold water to remove blood and then sterilized by boiling for several minutes in water containing 2 percent of washing soda. When facilities for boiling are not available, the cleaned instruments and needles may be immersed for 15 minutes or longer in a 2-percent lye solution, which must be freshly prepared each day and kept covered, as it deteriorates upon exposure to the air. After being removed from the lye solution, the needles may be dipped in a 2-percent compound solution of cresol, 2-percent formalin or 60- to 70-percent alcohol.

Natural Means of Transmission

Investigators working in various parts of the world have shown that anaplasmosts can be experimentally transmitted from diseased to healthy cattle by ticks, horseflies and mosquitoes. Additional research will doubtless reveal other vectors.

Several research workers have shown that the following 18 species of ticks are capable of transmitting anaplasmosis experimentally:

Scientific Name	*Common Name*
Boophilus annulatus	Cattle fever tick
B. decoloratus	Blue tick
B. microplus	None
Dermacentor albipictus	Winter tick
D. andersoni	Rocky Mountain spotted fever tick
D. occidentalis	Western dog tick
D. variabilis	American dog tick
Hyalomma lusitanicum	None
H. aegyptium	Bont-leg tick
Ixodes ricinus	Castor-bean tick
I. scapularis	Common shoulder tick
Ornithodorus lahorensis	None
Rhipicephalus appendiculatus	Common brown tick
R. bursa	Common brown tick
R. evertsi	Red-legged tick or red tick
R. sanguineus	Brown dog tick
R. simus	Black pitted tick
Argas persicus[4]	Chicken tick

[4] D.E. Howell and associates, Oklahoma Agricultural Experiment Station, unpublished data.

In his original work (1910), Theiler (25) showed that *Boophilus decoloratus* not only transmitted the disease called red water in South Africa but also anaplasmosis and that *Rhipicephalus simus* spread the same disease. In 1930 Rees (15) first experimentally incriminated *R. sanguineus* in this country as a carrier of anaplasmosis and the later transmitted the disease in the same manner with *Dermacentor andersoni, D. variabilis* and *Ixodes scapularis* (17).

In Du Toit's article on anaplasmosis (4), presented at the Twelfth International Veterinary Congress in 1934, be mentioned that several species of ticks had been reported by different workers as transmitting this disease. Rozeboom, Stiles and Moe (18) report transmission by *Dermacentor andersoni* and Stiles (24) records 17 ticks as vectors. From California, Boynton, Herms, Howell and Woods (1) reported in 1936 the successful transmission of anaplasmosis by *D. andersoni*, confirming the work of Rees. They also reported for the first time a new species, *D. albipictus* and a definite biological transmission of anaplasmosis by *D. occidentalis*. The disease was transmitted through both male and female ticks naturally infected with *D. andersoni* in 1938 by Sanborn, Stiles and Moe (20) and in 1940 hereditary transmission with the female of the species was accomplished by Howell, Stiles and Moe (8).

Horseflies also have been proved to be mechanical carriers of anaplasmosis. In many localities where the disease exists, large numbers of horseflies (tabanids) abound and home-made traps and commercial sprays are often employed to control them. In discussing these conditions, Sanborn *et al.* (19) state: "A study of field conditions, the prevalence of Tabanids, their occurrence, habits and distribution has been found to correspond closely to that of anaplasmosis. This is particularly true in swampy regions near ponds, inundated areas along rivers, lowlands of creeks and in wooded areas. These are the places where horseflies breed and develop and where the greatest annoyance to livestock occurs."

The first successful transmission of anaplasmosis by horseflies was accomplished by Sanborn, Stiles, Moe and Orr (21). Subsequently their findings were corroborated and summarized by Howell, Sanborn, Rozeboom, Stiles and Moe (7), who showed that seven species of horseflies can transmit the disease experimentally: *Tabanus sulcifrons, T. abactor, T. venustus, T. equalis, T. erythraeus, T. americanus* and *T. oklahomensis.*

In part the summary referred to states: "Fewer bites are required if the infecting animal is in the acute stage of the disease than if it is a carrier. Bites obtained five or more minutes after the infective feed were not able to transfer anaplasmosis to healthy animals." These findings may partly explain the sporadic nature of the disease and the apparent slowness of its spread.

In Florida in 1933 Sanders (22) incriminated *Tabanus fumipennis* and *Stomaxys calcitrans* as vectors and Morris, Martin and Oglesby (14), working in Louisiana, produced the disease from bites of *Tabanus atratus*.

Experiments conducted by Lotze and Yiengst (11) during the summer of 1941 at the Beltsville Research Center indicated conclusively that after feeding on an infected bull *Tabanus sulcifrons* transmitted anaplasmosis to three healthy cows within a period of 24 to 28 days. These large biting flies were of one of the seven species used by Sanborn *et al.* (Fig. 2.)

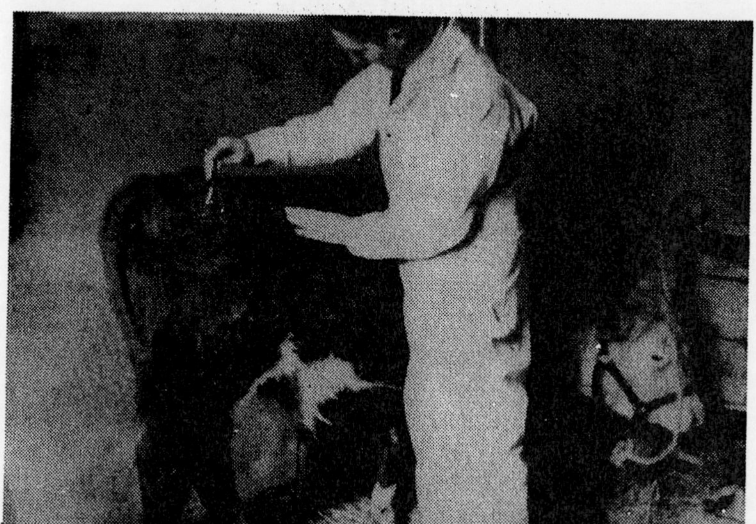

Fig. 2: A glass funnel is used to permit horseflies to feed on cattle in experiments on the transmissions of anaplasmosis at the Oklahoma Agricultural Experiment Station.

Since mosquitoes are known vectors of certain diseases, including malaria, yellow fever, fowl pox and equine sleeping sickness, these insects also were tested for their ability to transmit anaplasmosis.

Mosquitoes are often present during the anaplasmosis season in large numbers and cause considerable annoyance to cattle. The genus *Psorophora* often breeds in transient pools where cattle graze and since they are vicious biters, they were suspected of transmitting the disease. That they do so was proved by experimental feedings.

During the summer of 1940 Howell, Stiles and Moe (9) were the first workers to demonstrate the transmission of anaplasmosis by mosquitoes. In one instance 1,525 mosquitoes, *Psorophora columbiae* and *P. ciliata*, were fed on a cow with a clinical case of anaplasmosis and then allowed to feed on a healthy cow, which developed a typical case of anaplasmosis after 38 days. A second experiment, using three species of mosquitoes, *P. ciliata*, *P. columbiae* and *Aedes aegypti*, resulted in a positive case of anaplasmosis 58 days after the first feeding or 38 days after the last of 241 feedings.

Literature Cited

(1) BOYNTON, WILLIAM HUTCHINS, MERMS, WILLIAH B., HOWELL, D.E. and WOODS, GLADYS M. (1936). ANAPLASKOSIS TRANSMISSION BY THREE SPECIES OF TICKS IN CALIFORNIA. Amer. Vet. Med. Assoc. Jour. 88: 500-502.

(2) ______WOOD, F.W. and WOODS, GLADYS M. (1937). A NOTE ON TREATMENT OF ANAPLASMOSIS. North Amer. Vet. 18(5): 29-30.

(3) DIKMANS, G. (1988) ANAPLASMOSIS. V. THE NATURE OF ANAPLASMA. Amer. Vet. Med. Assoc. Jour. 88: 101-104.

(4) DUTOIT, P.J. (1934). ANAPLASMOSIS. 12th Internatl. Vet. Cong. Proc. 3: 325-345.

(5) DYKSTRA, R.R., LIENHARDT, H.F., PYLE, C.A. and FARLEY, H. (1938). STUDIES IN ANAPLASMOSIS. (Abstract) Expt. Sta. Rec. 79: 392.

(6) HILTS, W.H. (1928). ANAPLASMOSIS IN CATTLE FOLLOWING DEHORNING. Cornell Vet. 18: 330-332.

(7) HOWELL, D.E., SANBORN, C.E., ROZEBOOM, L E. and others (1941). THE TRANSMISSION OF ANAPLASMOSIS BY HORSEFLIES (TABANIDAE). Okla. Agr. Expt. Sta. Tech. Bul. T-11, 28 pp.

(8) ______STILES, GEO. W. and MOE, LEWIS H. (1941). THE HEREDITARY TRANSMISSION OF ANAPLASMOSIS BY DERMAOENTOR ANDERSONI STILES. Amer. Vet. Med. Assoc. Res. Jour. 2: 165-166.

(9) HOWELL, D.E., STILES, GEO. W. and MOE, LEWIS H. (1941). THE TRANSMISSION OF ANAPLASMOSIS BY MOSQUITOES (OULOIDAE). Amer. Vet. Med. Assoc. Jour. 99: 107-109.

(10) KOGER, R.B. (1941). WHOLE BLOOD IN THE TREATMENT OF ANAPLASMOSIS. Vet. Med. 36: 316-318, illus.

(11) LOTZE, JOHN C. and YIENGST, MABVIN J. (1941). MECHANICAL TRANSMISSION OF BOVINE ANAPLASMOSIS BY THE HORSEFLY TABANUS SULCIFRONS (MACQUART). Amer. Jour. Vet. Res., 2: 323-326, Illus.

(12) MOE, LEWIS H., STILES, GEO. W. and HOWELL, D.E. (1940). ANAPLASMOSIS TRANSMITTED BY TIPPING THE HORNS OF CATTLE. Amer. Vet. Med. Assoc. Jour. 97: 450-451.

(13) MOHLER, JOHN R. (1932). TICK FEVER. U. S. Dept. Agr. Farmers' Bul. 1625, 29 pp., illus. (Revised.)

(14) MORRIS, HARRY, MARTIN, J.A. and OGLESBY, W.T. (1936). AN ATTEMPT TO TRANSMIT ANAPLASMOSIS BY BITING FLIES. Amer. Vet. Med. Assoc. Jour. 89: 169-175.

(15) REES, CHARLES W. (1930). THE EXPERIMENTAL TRANSMISSION OF ANAPLASMOSIS BY RHIPICEPHALUS SANGUINEUS. North Amer. Vet. 2 (8): 17-20, illus.

(16) _______(1930). EXPERIMENTAL TRANSMISSION OF BOVINE ANAPLASMOSIS AND PIROPLASMOSIS BY MEANS OF AN INFECTED LANCET. North Amer. Vet. 2 (10): 17-20.

(17) _______(1934). TRANSMISSION OF ANAPLASMOSIS BY VARIOUS SPECIES OF TICKS. U.S. Dept. Agr. Tech. Bul. 418, 17 pp., illus.

(18) ROZEBOOM, LLOYD E., STILES, GEO. W. and MOE, LEWIS H. (1940). ANAPLASMOSIS TRANSMISSION BY DERMACENTOR ANDERSONI STILES. Jour. Parasitol. 26: 95-100.

(19) SANBORN, C.E., STILES, GEORGE W. and MOE, LEWIS H. (1932). PRELIMINARY EXPERIMENTS IN THE TRANSMISSION OF ANAPLASMOSIS BY HORSEFLIES. Okla. Agr. Expt. Sta. Bul. 204, 15 pp., illus.

(20) _______STILES, GEO. W. and MOE, LEWIS H. (1938). ANAPLASMOSIS TRANSMISSION BY NATURALLY INFECTED DERMACENTOR ANDERSONI MALE AND FEMALE TICKS. North Amer. Vet. 19 (1): 31-33.

(21) _______STILES, GEORGE W., MOE, LEWIS H. and ORR, HARRY W. (1930). TRANSMISSION OF ANAPLASMOSIS BY FLIES. In Okla. Agr. Expt. Sta. Rpt. 1926-30 (Research Leads to Farm Progress), pp. 254-264, illus.

(22) SANDERS, D.A. (1933). NOTES ON THE EXPERIMETNAL TRANSMISSION OF BOVINE ANAPLASMOSIS IN FLORIDA. Amer. Vet. Med. Assoc. Jour. 83: 799-805.

(23) STILES, GEO. W., JR. (1936). MECHANICAL TRANSMISSION OF ANAPLASMOSIS BY UNCLEAN INSTRUMENTS. North Amer. Vet. 17(6): 39-41.

(24) _______(1939). ANAPLASMOSIS IN CATTLE. U.S. Deptt. Agr. Cir. 154, 10 pp., illus. (Revised.)

(25) THEILES, A. (1910). ANAPLASMA MARGINALE, THE MARGINAL POINTS IN THE BLOOD OF CATTLE SUFFERING FBOM A SPECIFIC DISEASE. Transvaal Govt. Vet. Bact. Rpt., 1908-9: 7-64, illus.

(26) UNITED STATES BUREAU OF ANIMAL INDUSTRY. (1941). REPORT OF THE CHIEF OF THE BUREAU OF ANIMAL INDUSTRY 1941. 92 pp.

(27) VAWTER, L.R. and RECORDS, EDWARD (1926). RECENT STUDIES ON ICTERO-HEMOGLOBINURIA OF CATTLE. Amer. Vet. Med. Assoc. Jour. 68: 494-513, illus.

Chapter 11

CATTLE SCAB AND ITS CONTROL

Rudolph Snyder[1]

[1] *Rudolph Snyder is Senior Veterinarian and Assistant Chief of the Interstate Inspection Division, Bureau of Animal Industry.*

Common scab of cattle, once widespread and serious in this country, has been almmost eradicated, but sarcoptic scab, once rare, is now becoming a real menace. These and the two other types of cattle scab are discussed in this article.

In his annual report for 1902, the Chief of the Bureau of Animal Industry referred to numerous inquiries about a disease commonly known as Texas itch. As the disease appears to have been more prevalent in other sections of the Country than in Texas, it seems strange that this name was applied to it. At that time the disease was apparently fairly common among the range cattle of the West and Northwest and it had also been heard of in other parts of the country. Investigation showed that the condition was scabies, a contagious skin disease commonly known as scab, mange or itch, caused by insectlike parasites called mites.

There are four species of the scabies parasite which affect cattle and they belong to four different genera-*Psoroptes, Sarcoptes, Chorioptes* and *Demodex*. The psoroptic mites, which cause common scab, live in groups or colonies on the surface of the skin and the lesions or damage to tissues they cause, spread in all directions from the spot first affected. The sarcoptic mites, which cause what is known in some regions as barn itch, bore into the skin, each female making a separate gallery in which she lays her eggs. The chorioptic mites live in groups on the surface of the skin and usually remain localized on the legs or tail with little or no tendency to spread. The demodectic mites are microscopic in size and are more like worms than typical mites; they live in the hair follicles and sebaceous (sweat and oil) glands and cause smooth spherical swellings or pustules, in the skin.

Psoroptic or Common, Scab

The mites causing psoroptic or common, scab of cattle were encountered throughout the range and semirange States in the early 1900's. Although not so dangerous a disease as sarcoptic scab, psoroptic scab caused more extensive losses to the livestock industry because of its greater prevalence. It occasionally occurs on cattle in farming communities in various parts of the country, and, unless properly treated, it causes great losses through reduction in weight, failure of young stock to thrive and gain weight normally and an increase in the death rate especially among cattle in a state of poor nutrition and low vitality when they are exposed to inclement weather.

The mites that cause common cattle scab are small white or yellowish parasites known technically as *Psoroptes equi bovis* or perhaps more often as *Psoroptes communis bovis*. The female when full grown measures about one-fortieth and the male about one-fiftieth of an inch in length. They are visible to the naked eye, especially when placed on a dark background. The entire life cycle is passed on the body of a host animal. Each female may deposit 15 to 24 eggs, which hatch after 3 or 4 days' incubation. The young mites reach maturity and mate and the females of the new generation deposit eggs in 10 to 12 days.

The mites may attack any part of the body that is thickly covered with hair. The first symptom of the disease is usually an intense itching of the skin on the withers, on the top of the neck just in front of the withers or around the root of the tail. From these points the lesions spread over the back and sides and, unless checked, may involve practically the entire body.

The most certain diagnosis consists in demonstrating the presence of the parasite that causes the disease. This may be done by scraping the outer edges of the infected areas with a blunt-edged knife and transferring the scrapings to a smooth black surface, such as a piece of black paper. Spreading the scrapings in the warm sun or near artificial heat usually causes the mites to become active and they can be seen as minute, gray, moving bodies against the dark background. Well-advanced cases of scab are usually easy to diagnose, but the disease should never be allowed to reach this stage; in the early stages it yields readily to proper treatment, but if allowed to spread it will entail heavy losses.

The transmissibility of the disease is not limited to any one season of the year, although cattle on green, succulent feed and in a thriving condition seldom contract scab. In fact, in the spring, when infected cattle are turned out on green grass, the old coat of hair is shed and the disease often seems to have been cured. It will usually break out again, however, with the coming of cold, stormy weather.

Although the infected animal is the most important factor in spreading cattle mites, infected premises should not be overlooked. Owing to the varying conditions that may affect the ability of the mite and its eggs to remain alive when separated from a host, it is impossible to state definitely how long premises may remain infectious after the removal of the cattle. Hence, it is advisable to clean and disinfect all infected sheds, barns, yards or small inclosures thoroughly before using them for clean or dipped cattle. There are a number of cresylic disinfectants which when diluted in accordance with instructions on the container are suitable for this purpose.

Control Measures

The only rational way to treat cattle scabies is to use some external application that will kill the parasites without injuring the animals. Dipping is the method most commonly used to accomplish this. It consists in immersing the animals in a medicated liquid that will thoroughly wet the entire surface of the body and kill the parasites. It is the only method recognized by the Bureau of Animal Industry in the official treatment of scabby cattle because it is the most practical and effective. Dipping plants are usually arranged so that the cattle enter one end of a vat filled with the dip, swim through its and leave the vat at the opposite end. The dips commonly used by the Bureau of Animal Industry and permitted for use in official dipping of cattle for scabies are lime-sulfur solution and a nicotine solution.

The stages in the life cycle of the mite have an important bearing on the interval which should elapse between treatments for common scab. Dipping properly done will kill the mites but cannot be depended upon to destroy an the eggs and the animals should be dipped a second time before the newly hatched mites have had time to develop and deposit eggs. Practical experience has shown that the interval between the first and second dippings should be 10 to 12 days, although in some instances this may be safely extended to a maximum of 14 days.

During 1903 some preliminary inspections and dippings were carried out and in 1904 regulations were issued which placed in quarantine that part of the United States lying west of the Mississippi River and the eastern boundary of Minnesota. This quarantine specified the manner in which cattle could be shipped to other States from the area. In 1905 the quarantine was modified to include only those areas in which the disease was prevalent. During that year a large force was placed in the field by the Bureau of Animal Industry to make inspections and supervise the dipping of exposed and infected animals. From 1904 to 1911 cattle scabies seemed to be increasing rapidly in many States, but after 1911 the effects of the systematic eradication measures carried on by the Bureau in cooperation with the livestock sanitary officials of the various States became apparent. The common variety of cattle scabies has been practically eradicated and at the present time no territory is under Federal quarantine for this disease.

Sarcoptic Scab

Sarcoptic scab or mange or barn itch, is found more or less frequently on both farm and range cattle throughout the country. Owing to its comparative rarity, it was not formerly considered of much importance in the United States, but during the last few years it has been increasing and must now be considered a major problem. The disease is more serious than common scab because it is more severe in its effects and more difficult to eradicate. It sometimes develops in purebred cattle and animals from purebred herds may carry the infection although they may not show visible symptoms of scabies at the time they are shipped. Purebred bulls of the beef breeds seem to be especially susceptible and may be an important factor in spreading the disease. The breeder of purebred cattle who supplies bulls for building up range and farm herds finds his business very nearly ruined when sarcoptic scabies develops in his herd. In dairy herds it may seriously affect milk production and throw the balance on the wrong side of the ledger. The disease can be eradicated, however and if proper methods are adopted before it reaches an advanced stage the losses can be reduced to a minimum.

The parasites *Sarcoptes scabiei* var. *caprae*, which cause sarcoptic scab, resemble in a general way the common scab mites. The entire life cycle is passed on the body of the host animal, but the sarcoptic mites do not remain on the surface; they penetrate the outer layer of the skin and excavate burrows or galleries in which mating occurs and the eggs are laid. When egg laying is completed the female dies in her burrow.

The mites prefer locations where the skin is tender and the hair is thin. In the early stages of the disease the lesions are usually found on the inner surfaces of the thighs, the under side of the neck or brisket or around the root of the tall. From these parts the entire surface of the body may become involved.

Sarcoptic scab is transmissible from one species of animal to another and also from animals to man. Sarcoptic mites of the horse, sheep, goat and cat may live on cattle, while those of the horse, dog and hog are known to be readily transmissible to man; but ordinarily, when one species contracts the contagion from another species, the mites live only a short time on the newly infected animal. Sarcoptic scab of cattle is contagious to all classes of cattle and is transmitted by direct contact with animals or objects that are carriers of the mites.

It is evident, therefore, that all stables and small enclosures occupied by mangy cattle and all implements and coverings, such as curry-combs, brushes and blankets, should be cleaned and disinfected before they are used for clean or dipped cattle. The cleaning and disinfection should be done in the same manner as for common scab.

Probably on account of their burrowing habit, sarcoptic mites are much more difficult to eradicate than the common scab mites. The dips recommended for the latter will kill sarcoptic mites if the liquid comes in contact with them, but it may not reach all the mites at one application. Persistent, thorough and frequent application of the dip will effect a cure, however, especially if all infected parts are scrubbed well with a brush and soaked with dipping solution just prior to the first dipping. Experience has shown that four dippings in either a lime-sulfur or a nicotine dip will cure sarcoptic scab in cattle. The interval between dippings should be 6 to 10 days.

One dipping in crude petroleum usually cures sarcoptic scab, as it seems to destroy the eggs as well as the mites. A serious drawback to its use as a dip for cattle, however, is that in some cases it is injurious to the animals.

Chorioptic or Symbiotic, Scab

Chorioptic or symbiotic, scab occurs occasionally in cattle, but it is of less importance than either of the two varieties already described. It is caused by a mite called *Chorioptes bovis,* which under a high-power magnifying glass closely resembles the common scab mite. Though it usually spreads very slowly, the disease is contagious to all classes of cattle. The mites live on the surface of the skin and produce lesions resembling those of common scab. The lesions are usually found on the tail or legs and generally remain localized. For practical purposes it is not necessary to distinguish between chorioptic and common scab, because the same treatment is recommended for both.

Demodectic Mange

Until about 1923 demodectic or follicular, mange of cattle, caused by the mite called *Demodex bovis,* was not often recognized in the United States. Owing to the damage to leather caused by demodectic mange lesions, however, an investigation was made in 1927 to determine the extent of the disease and numerous cases were reported from 14 States, most of which were in old cows of the dairy breeds. The lesions of demodectic mange in cattle appear as nodules or small lumps, most often in the skin of the neck, shoulders, breast and dew-lap and sometimes in other parts of the body. Demodectic mange may progress rapidly on an animal until the nodules appear nearly everywhere in the skin or there may be no alteration in the number and size of the nodules during a period of several years. Ordinarily the disease does not spread rapidly from an infected animal to others in the herd, but precautions should be taken to prevent possible spread by isolating infected animals. There is no known practical remedy for demodectic mange in cattle, although frequent dippings delay the progress of the disease and may cure mild cases.

Chapter 12

TAPEWORM AND ROUNDWORM PARASITES OF CATTLE

Dale A. Porter[1]

[1] *Dale A. Porter is Associate Parasitologist, Regional Animal Disease Research Laboratory, Auburn, Ala., Bureau of Animal Industry.*

Seventy or more species of tapeworms and roundworms infest cattle, some causing serious losses. Here are facts about the more important, including methods of prevention and treatment. The article on worm parasites of sheep should also be read by those interested, practically and scientifically, in cattle worms.

Tapeworm and roundworm parasites reported to affect cattle throughout the world comprise over 70 different species. Although some species occur infrequently and others are comparatively harmless to their bovine hosts, some exact a heavy annual toll from the beef dairy industries. Losses are due to deaths from gross parasitism, lowered vitality and resultant poor growth and performance and condemnation, in the course of meat inspection, of carcasses or edible parts as a result of invasion by parasites.

Members of these two groups of parasites–tapeworms and roundworms–vary considerably in their location, structure and harmfulness.

The cestodes or tapeworms, of cattle are found as adults in the intestine and as larval forms in the muscles, liver, lungs and other viscera. The adults are elongated, flattened worms consisting of a head and a chain of segments, each having both male and female reproductive organs and terminal segments containing mature eggs. The larval forms, commonly referred to as bladder worms because they resemble a bladder in shape, are intermediate asexual stages of tapeworms that live as adults in the intestines of man and other animals. The bladder worms vary in diameter from one-fourth inch in the case of the beef bladder worm (*Cysticercus bovis*) to as much as 6 inches in the case of the hydatid cysts (*Echinococcus granulosus*).

Although migration is common during development, the adult roundworms or nematodes, to be discussed in this article occur in the digestive tract or lungs. Some roundworms, the lungworms and stomach worms, for example, are named for the location in which they are commonly found. The roundworms are elongated, cylindrical, unsegmented worms and may be characterized as threadlike or hairlike. The sexes are generally separate and the males are usually smaller than the females.

Significant facts about the more common tapeworm and roundworm parasites of cattle and their control are discussed briefly in the following pages. The parasites of cattle are closely related to and in some instances specifically identical with, those occurring in sheep and from the standpoint of present knowledge more facts have been determined concerning parasitism in the latter host.

Cestoda or Tapeworms

Adult Tapeworms in the Intestine

Cattle in this country are known to harbor two species of tapeworms, *Moniezia benedeni* and *M. expansa*, both of which are common and sometimes serious pests of sheep also. The worms are whitish to yellowish in color and when mature may be several feet long and as much as three-fourths of an inch wide. The life history of *M. benedeni* is probably similar to that of *M. expansa*. The latter is transmitted by means of a tiny grass mite prevalent on pastures, particularly in damp areas. The mites eat the tapeworm eggs passed in the manure of cattle or sheep harboring the adult worms. The egg develops into a larval tapeworm within the mite and when the mite is eaten by cattle the larval tapeworm is digested out and settles down in the small intestine, eventually reaching the adult stage (*8, 17, 18*).[2] As the worm grows, the terminal segments become filled with eggs that escape into the intestine and pass out in the droppings. The mature terminal segments, either individually or several together, are occasionally seen in the droppings of calves, particularly when they have diarrhoea and this aids in diagnosing the parasites.

It is generally believed that tapeworms do less damage in cattle than in sheep. Older animals are seldom affected, but young calves may harbor several of the worms, which may cause enough intestinal irritation to interfere with digestion and thus make the calves weak and unthrifty.

Tapeworm Cysts in the Liver and Other Viscera

The hydatid (*Echinococcus granulosus*) and the thin-necked bladder worm (*Cysticercus tenuicollis*) are the intermediate stages of two tapeworms, *Taenia echinococcus* and *T. hydatigena*, which as adults are parasites in the intestines of dogs, wolves and other canines. Closely related zoologically, their life histories are essentially similar. The canine hosts acquire the adult worms as a result of eating the cysts in dead animals or in offal from slaughtered animals. Cattle in turn acquire the larvae as a result of swallowing tapeworm eggs eliminated in the droppings of parasitized canines that have access to cattle pastures. The eggs hatch in the small intestine and the embryo enters the intestinal wall, to be distributed by the blood stream to the preferred sites of development in the body. These bladder worms are found more frequently in sheep and swine than in cattle.

The hydatid forms fluid-filled, tumorlike cysts ranging up to several inches in diameter in the liver, lungs and other organs. The bovine host is seldom suspected of harboring these parasites during life, although there may be pulmonary or digestive disturbances, depending upon the location of the cysts. Even the presence of large numbers of cysts which may have caused extensive tissue destruction is usually discovered only at slaughter.

The thin-necked bladder worm, *Cysticercus tenuicollis*, occurs embedded in the liver, attached to other abdominal organs or free in

---

[2] Italic numbers in parentheses refer to Literature Cited.

the body cavity. The parasite looks like a sac full of clear liquid, usually about 1 inch in diameter. As in the case of the hydatid, the occurrence of this parasite in cattle cannot be diagnosed during life. A few bladder worms apparently have little or no effect on the host and large numbers involving extensive liver damage by the immature larval form, as described in the case of sheep, have not been observed in cattle.

Tapeworm Cysts in the Muscles

The beef tapeworm (*Taenia saginata*), in the adult stage a parasite of man, occurs in cattle in the larval or bladder worm, stage and is then known as *Cysticercus bovis.*

The condition in cattle caused by this worm is commonly referred to as beef measles. The cysticercus consists of a head, a neck and a fluid-filled bladder within which the head and neck are inserted or sheathed. The worms appear as oval white vesicles about the size of a pea and occur throughout the muscles of the body but most frequently in the heart, muscles of mastication, diaphragm and tongue. The life cycle involves an alternation between the two hosts, human beings and cattle. Infection of man is brought about by eating the bladder worm in raw or incompletely cooked beef; cattle in turn acquire the larvae as a result of swallowing the tapeworm eggs with drinking water or forage that has become contaminated with the excreta of the human tapeworm carrier. The small larvae hatch from the eggs in the stomach. Upon reaching the intestine they burrow into the gut wall and are carried by the blood stream, aided probably by their own movements, to various locations in the body. Development to the infective cystic stage has been estimated to take from 7 to 18 weeks. Numerous cases of cysticercosis or measles, detected under Federal meat-inspection procedure have been traced back to contacts with human carriers on farms and ranches.

Usually there are no definite symptoms associated with measles in cattle and diagnosis depends on finding the cysts in the animals on post mortem examination. The economic importance of the parasite is in its relationship to human health. On account of the danger to human health from eating measly beef, precautions are taken to detect the parasite in beef carcasses through Federal and other equally thorough meat-inspection procedures.

Nematoda or Roundworms

Lungworms

Lungworms of cattle (*Dictyocalus viviparus*) are white, threadlike worms 2 to 3 inches long. They inhabit chiefly the medium-sized and smaller bronchial tubes of the lungs. The female worms produce large numbers of eggs which usually hatch in the air passages, liberating larvae which are coughed up, swallowed and eliminated in the feces. Sometimes the coughed-up eggs hatch in the stomach or intestines, but they often pass unhatched from the host, particularly when there is severe diarrhoea.

Under favorable conditions the larvae eliminated with the feces develop to the infective stage in about a week. The infective larvae tend to migrate on grass in warm, wet weather and are taken in with the grass by grazing cattle. The course of development following ingestion of the larvae is believed to be similar to that of the lungworm of sheep. (*Dictyocaulus filaria*). In this case the larvae penetrate the intestinal wall and reach the lymph glands, from which they are eventually carried to the lungs. The writer has observed that cattle lungworms mature in 3 to 4 weeks, at which time larvae appear in the feces and that the worms are apparently capable of living 2 to 4 months within the host.

The worms and their eggs and larvae irritate the lung tissue, producing local inflammation which is manifested by the production of considerable frothy mucus. The extent of the damage to the functioning lung depends largely on the number of parasites present and the age and condition of the host; the parasites occur much more frequently in calves than in mature cattle. In light or moderate cases no symptoms are shown, with the possible exception of an occasional dry cough and poor condition. If the invasion is extensive there are frequent coughing spells, difficult breathing and progressive weakness. The cases that usually prove fatal are those in which there is extensive involvement of the lungs, particularly as a result of the secondary invasion of bacteria. Such instances are characterized by shallow breathing with the mouth open and the tongue protruded (Fig. 1). Death results from exhaustion of suffocation brought on by mechanical blocking of the air passages by worms and the accompanying discharge of mucus and pus.

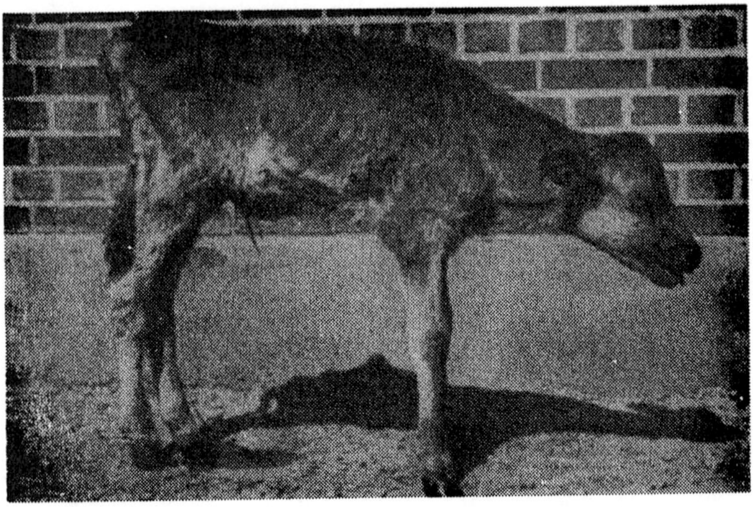

Fig. 1: A 2-mouth-old calf with lungworm disease. Note the open mouth.

Stomach Worms

Three species of roundworms (*Haemonchus contortus, Ostertagia ostertagi* and *Trichostrongylus axei*) are common parasites in the abomasum or fourth stomach, of cattle. Of these the first is the best known and is commonly referred to as the stomach worm or twisted wireworm.

The roundworm *Haemonchus contortus* is 1½ inch to 1½ inches long and about as thick as an ordinary pin. The female worms produce large numbers of eggs, which pass out in the feces and hatch in a few hours under favorable conditions. The larvae, hatching from the egg, undergo two molts, reaching the infective stage in about 4 or 5 days.

The infective larvae retain the last molt or skin and, thus ensheathed, are very resistant to cold and long periods of dryness. When there is rain or dew these larvae crawl up on blades of grass, with which they are swallowed by grazing cattle. The worms become mature in the stomach in 3 to 4 weeks.

Haemonchus contortus apparently affects cattle in the same way that it does sheep, although there may be some differences in the degree of cross transmission between the two hosts. According to Clunies Ross (*5*), lambs may be parasitized readily by *H. contortus* of either ovine (sheep) or bovine origin, whereas calves are parasitized with difficulty by *H. contortus* of bovine origin. As in the case of sheep, younger animals are the ones most seriously affected, although losses may occur occasionally along 3-year-olds (*12*). Among the common symptoms produced by this parasite are loss of flesh, general weakness and anemia. The anemic condition, due to impoverishment of the blood from the bloodsucking habit of the worms, may be recognized by the paleness of the skin and mucous membranes of the mouth and eyes and the edema or watery swelling, known as bottle jaw, which often develops under the jaw (Fig. 2). The latter condition is particularly noticeable after the animal has been driven or otherwise strenuously exercised. Diarrhoea has also been considered as symptomatic, but the writer has not observed it in calves showing other clinical symptoms in experimental infections with stomach worms.

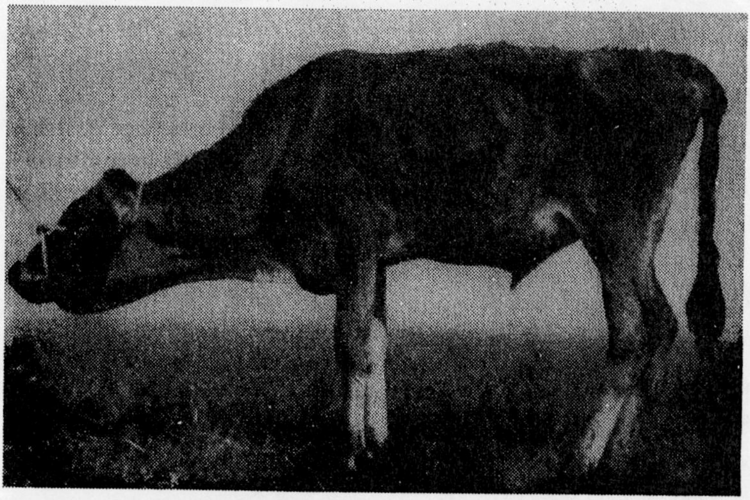

Fig. 2: A yearling steer with stomach worm disease. Note the submaxillary edema, or bottle jaw.

Ostertagia ostertagi, another parasite of the fourth stomach of cattle, is also occasionally found in sheep. A small hairlike worm, slightly over one-fourth of an inch in length, it may often be overlooked. From what is known, its life history is similar to that of *Haemonchus contortus*. The infective larvae ingested with food reach the abomasum and there penetrate into the mucous membrane. Development to maturity takes place in small cystic nodules or lumps, produced by the host in an attempt to overcome the invading larvae. Upon reaching maturity the adult worms escape into the stomach leaving the abandoned nodules to degenerate. The resulting patchy erosion may be detected as small white circumscribed areas on the stomach lining. The wall of the stomach may also be extremely thickened and swollen in severe cases.

In some sections of the United States, notably in the West, this parasite may replace *Haemonchus contortus* in importance. Stiles (*15*) considered it to be the chief factor in a severe outbreak of verminous disease in Texas cattle. Several outbreaks of verminous gastritis (inflammation of the stomach) due to this parasite have been described. In outbreaks among yearling animals in which there were several deaths, the symptoms were emaciation, anemia, rough coat and a diarrhoea of varying intensity (*1, 3*). Submaxillary edema (bottle jaw) similar to that seen in cattle haemonchosis has also been reported.

Of the nematode parasites found in the stomachs of cattle, the third species, *Trichostrongylus axei*, is the least specific to a particular host. Large numbers of these parasites, which produce gastritis, have been observed in horses as well as cattle and other ruminants. Available evidence also indicates that this nematode may be transferred from one host species to another (*4, 16, 20*).

The parasites themselves are very slender and only about one-fifth of an inch or less in length. They are found on or in the mucous lining of the stomach and detecting them usually depends on microscopical examination of scrapings made from the stomach lining. The details of the life history are not fully known but it has been determined that the host is parasitized by swallowing the infective larvae that develop in the feces of other animals harboring the parasite (*4*).

Injuries to the bovine stomach consist of patchy gastritis in which the lining of the stomach is thickened and thrown into folds

(2). Such symptoms as severe diarrhoea and loss of condition have been associated with the presence of large numbers of these roundworms.

Cooperids

Three species of small nematodes (*Cooperia punctata*, *C. pectinata* and *C. oncophora*), known collectively as cooperids, occur in cattle in the United States. *C. punctata* has a rather general distribution, having been encountered frequently in both the Northern and the Southern States. *C. pectinata* is prevalent mainly in the South and *C. oncophora* is more prevalent in the North (*6*).

The adult worms are found on or imbedded in the mucous membrane, predominantly in the upper portion of the small intestine. Hairlike in thickness and about one-quarter inch long, the worms may be overlooked in a superficial examination. The development and transmission of these species are similar to those of the large stomach worm, *Haemonchus contortus*.

It is quite apparent that the cooperids are capable of producing extensive intestinal inflammation in calves. Descriptions given by Hung (*7*) and Dikmans (*6*) indicate that *Cooperia punctata* penetrates the intestinal mucous membrane and the layer beneath, producing a destructive inflammation that is particularly severe where the worms are numerous. Such lesions or tissue injuries appear on examination as accumulations of white or yellow cheesy material (*11*). Seriously affected animals have more or less persistent diarrhoea and become emaciated and anemic as the disease progresses.

By reason of their widespread distribution and common occurrence these roundworms may be responsible for more cases of intestinal inflammation and unthriftiness in young cattle than is now generally recognized.

Hookworms

The cattle hookworm, called scientifically *Bunostomum phlebotomum*, belongs to the same family as the hookworms of other animals, including man and shares the familial reputation of being a bloodsucker. A prevalent parasite of young cattle, this worm occurs normally in the upper small intestine, but it may invade the fourth stomach in small numbers and attach itself to the gastric mucous membrane. The worms attain a length of three-fourths of an inch to an inch and appear pinkish white in the intestine. The eggs of the female hookworm pass from the host in the droppings, hatch and develop to the infective stage. According to Schwartz (*14*), they hatch in about 96 hours under laboratory conditions at a temperature of 70° to 80° F. The larvae undergo two molts, the third or infective stage completing a cycle of development that required a minimum of 7 days. The infective larvae may be swallowed by cattle while grazing or penetrate the skin and develop to maturity upon reaching the intestine. The details of migration of the lavae following skin penetration are lacking. Probably the route is similar to that of the sheep hookworm (*B. trigonocephalum*), the larvae of which penetrate the skin, migrate to the lungs, presumably by way of the blood stream and thence to the intestine by way of the windpipe, mouth and gullet (*10*).

As is common with the hookworms, the adult is provided with mouth parts capable of attaching it to the intestinal mucous membrane. Aside from sucking blood directly from the host, the small lacerations produced by the mouth of the worm may be left bleeding as the worm moves from one place of attachment to another. This species, when present in large numbers, is capable of producing clinical symptoms similar to those produced by the stomach worm, *Haemonchus contortus*. According to Roberts (*12*), the disease runs a well-marked course of weakness, emaciation, intermittent diarrhoea and progressive anemia in which the red-cell count may be reduced as much as 75 percent in severe cases.

Nodular Worms

Unlike the intestinal worms discussed previously, the nodular worm, which is known as *Oesophagostonum radiatum*, is found in the large intestine and cecum. This worm is about five-eighths of an inch long and white in color. The eggs of the female are passed with the feces and larvae are hatched that undergo some development on the ground similar to that of the stomach worm, *Haemonchus coniortus*. The infective larvae swallowed by cattle enter the intestinal wall for a period of development and later migrate to the lumen of the intestine to develop to maturity.

The larval parasite and resulting secondary bacterial invasion cause the formation of nodules which, particularly after degenerations to a cheesy state, may be mistaken by inexperienced persons for the lesions of tuberculosis. Although the nodules may be encountered in the bovine omentum (a fold of the lining of the abdominal cavity), they are usually restricted to the posterior (rear) portion of the small intestine and to the large intestine and cecum. These nodules are usually somewhat smaller than those caused by a related species, *Oesophagostomum columbianum*, in sheep and the general effects of the parasite in cattle are believed to be somewhat less severe. Such symptoms as anemia, scouring and emaciation have been correlated with gross parasitism and because of the permanent nature of the nodules, recovery may be slow.

General Measures for Control

Control measures for any parasite depend on complete knowledge of its life history. Studies of the developmental stages usually reveal one in which the parasite is vulnerable to natural or man-made barriers and in which the life cycle may be broken. As research on parasites of cattle continues, control measures should be found which, if not capable of eradicating parasitism, certainly will be instrumental in reducing its toll.

Some general recommendations for the control of the more common tapeworm and roundworm parasites are given below:

Adult tapeworms in the intestine

The transmission of these tapeworms (*Moniezia* species) involves certain free-living mites as intermediate hosts, but as yet too little is known about their life history or habits to make full recommendations for control. However, since young stock is most often affected, pastures known to be a source of infection should be closed to calves.

Tapeworm cysts of the liver and other viscera

The control of hydatids and thin-necked bladder worms, both intermediate stages of adult tapeworms in canines, depends on some barrier between dogs and cattle. To effect this barrier, stray dogs and other canines should be kept off farms and suppressed by appropriate measures. Also, dogs belonging on the premises should be kept free of tapeworms by suitable remedies. As a precaution against infection of dogs with tapeworms, the viscera of slaughtered cattle, sheep and hogs should be disposed of in such a manner as to be inaccessible to the dogs.

Tapeworm cysts of the muscles

To prevent cattle from acquiring the cysticercus of the human tapeworm, *Taenia saginata,* care should be taken that human feces are not disposed of in such a manner as to contaminate the feed and drinking water of the cattle. Prevention of tapeworm in the human being is simple and effective: Cook beef thoroughly.

Roundworm parasites

In view of the similarity in the development of the free-living stages of the commonly important gastrointestinal roundworms and lungworms of cattle, preventive measures are in general applicable for all species concerned. Any control measures should be set up primarily to reduce the chances that calves and yearlings will become seriously parasitized, since young cattle are the most susceptible.

As moisture favors the development of the eggs and larvae of roundworms, well-drained pastures are preferable and low, wet areas should be avoided until they are drained. Drinking water should be supplied from wells or flowing streams, preferably in troughs raised above the ground. Pastures that it is impractical to drain should be used only for mature cattle.

Pastures should not be overstocked and rotation, as often as available forage permits, is highly desirable, since free-living stages of the parasites in a contaminated field will largely succumb in the absence for a sufficient time, of susceptible hosts.

Young animals being most susceptible to parasitism, calves should be kept as much as possible away from the older stock and the contaminated pastures and quarters where the latter have been confined. As a precaution against further spread of parasitism, any affected cattle should be isolated from the held for special treatment. Sanitation and good feeding will sometimes stop losses from parasitism even if no medicinal treatment is given.

Medicinal Treatment

Owing to the similarity of the effects of parasitism in cattle and in sheep the medicinal control of the tapeworm and roundworm parasites of cattle has followed closely the treatments recommended for sheep. In few instances, however, has the efficacy of the drugs been determined by critical tests on cattle; recommendations for their use are based largely on clinical data or the performance of the drugs on related worms in sheep.

A 1-percent solution of copper sulfate has been used for the control of the stomach worm *Haemonchus contortus*. This solution is given as a drench in doses of the following sizes: Calves, 3½ to 4 fluid ounces; yearlings, 6 fluid ounces; 2-year-old and older cattle, 12 to 16 fluid ounces. The addition of 1 ounce of 40-percent nicotine sulfate to a gallon of 1-percent copper sulfate administered in doses of the same sizes as above has also been recommended as a treatment for stomach worms, hookworms and tapeworms (*Moniezia* species). Monnig (*9*) reports that a mixture composed of 30 cubic centimeters of 40-percent nicotine sulfate and 30 grams of copper sulfate in 1,800 cubic centimeters of water has given satisfactory results against the tapeworms (*Moniezia*) and stomach worms (*Haemonchus*) in cattle in the field. The mixture is given at the rate of 30 cubic centimeters to each 50 pounds of live weight, with a maximum of 90 cubic centimeters for animals under 2 years of age and 120 to 150 cubic centimeters, according to size, for those over 2 years old. Crude castor oil is recommended as a purgative to follow this treatment for tapeworms.

Some investigators recommend tetrachlorethylene as a medicinal control for stomach worms, hookworms and the small intestinal roundworms (*Cooperia* species). This drug may be administered in capsules or as a drench in an emulsion consisting of equal parts of the drug and mineral oil. The dosage of tetrachlorethylene recommended is 10 to 15 cubic centimeters for calves 2 to 4 months old and up to 25 to 30 cubic centimeters for animals 12 to 18 months old (*13*). The tetrachlolethylene emulsion may be given immediately following the introduction of about 2 cubic centimeters of a 5-percent copper sulfate solution into the mouth (*2*). Recent critical tests (*19*) supplemented by clinical data indicate that phenothiazine may have considerable promise as an anthelmintic for the removal of stomach worms, hookworms and nodular worms. On the basis of available data, a dose of 20 grams per 100 pounds of live weight, with a maximum individual dose of 60 grams, administered in capsules, is suggested.

Treatment for parasites outside the gastrointestinal tract is unsuccessful. There are no medicinal agents for the removal of tapeworm cysts and although various chemicals have been administered by inhalation or injection into the windpipe for the removal of lung-worms, none has shown effectiveness. Lungworm cases are probably best treated by removing the animals from pasture to clean sanitary quarters and supplying liberal quantities of feed.

While parasitism may be suspected in young cattle in unthrifty condition, malnutrition or other conditions may be present, if not actually responsible. Animals in a weakened condition may react unfavorably to medication and it is therefore advisable to obtain competent diagnosis and advice before resorting to treatment.

In treating young cattle for parasites it is advisable to treat not only the animals that are seriously affected but also the rest of the herd, since any parasites remaining in the herd become a source of reinfection. Following treatment the animals should if possible be removed to fresh pastures.

Literature Cited

(1) ACKERT, JAMES E. and MULDOON, WILLIAM E. (1920). STRONGYLOSIS (OSTERTAGIA) IN CATTLE. Amer. Vet. Med: Assoc. Jour. 58: 138-146, illus.

(2) BAKER, DONALD W. (1939). A NEW SYSTEM OF ANTHELMINTIC CONTROL FOR GASTRO-INTESTINAL PARASITES OF RUMINANTS. Cornell Vet. 29: 192-197, illus.

(3) BARGER, E.H. (1927). OSTERTAGIA OSTERTAGI IN CALIFORNIA CATTLE, WITH COPPER SULPHATE AN APPARENTLY SUCCESSFUL THERAPEUTIC. Amer. Vet. Med. Assoc. Jour. 71: 560-567, illus.

(4) BRITTON, JOHN W. (1939). TRICHOSTRONGYLOSIS IN EQUINES. Cornell Vet. 29: 322-330.

(5) CLUNIES ROSS, I. (1931). THE HOST SPECIFICITY OF HAEMONCHUS CONTORTUS OF SHEEP AND CATTLE. Austral. Jour. Expt. Biol. and Med. Sci. 8: 217-224.

(6) DIKMANS, G. (1939). PARASITIC ENTERITIS IN CALVES. Vet. Med. 34: 28-30, illus.

(7) HUNG, SEE-LU (1926). THE PATHOLOGY OF COOPERIA PUNCTATA INFESTATION IN CALVES. North Amer. Vet. 7 (3): 33-36, illus.

(8) KRULL, WENDELL H. (1939). ON THE LIFE HISTORY OF MONIEZIA EXPANSA AND CITTOTAENIA SP. (CESTODA: ANOPLOCEPHALIDAE). Helminthol. Soc. Wash. Proc. 6: 10-11.

(9) MONNIG, H.O. (1937). ON THE TOXICITY OF NICOTINE FOR SHEEP AND THE USE OF THE NICOTINE-BLUESTONE DRENCH FOR WORMS IN RUMINANTS. Rev. de Med. Trop. Parisitol. 3: 3-10.

(10) ORTLEPP, R.J. (1939). OBSERVATIONS ON THE LIFE-HISTORY OF BUNOSTOMUM TRIGONOCEPHALUM, A HOOKWORM OF SHEEP AND GOATS. Onderstepoort Jour. Vet. Sci. and Anim. Indus. 12: 305-318, illus.

(11) RANSOM, [B.H.] (1920). INTESTINAL LESIONS IN CALVES DUE TO COOPERIA PUNCTATA. Jour. Parasitol. 7: 96.

(12) ROBERTS, F.H.S. (1939). THE GASTRO-INTESTINAL HELMINTHS OF CATTLE IN QUEENSLAND: THEIR DISTRIBUTION AND PATHOGENIC IMPORTANCE. Roy. Soc. Queensland Proc. (1938) 50: 46-54, illus.

(13) ______(1940). PARASITIC WORM DISEASES OF CATTLE. Queensland Dept. Agr. and Stock, Div. Ent. and Plant Pathol. Advisory Leaflet 26, 20 pp., illus.

(14) SCHWARTZ, BENJAMIN (1924). PREPARASITIC STAGES IN THE LIFE HISTORY OF THE CATTLE HOOKWORM (BUSTOMUM PHLEBOTOMUM). Jour. Agr. Res. 29: 451-458, illus.

(15) STILES, CH. WARDELL (1901). VERMINOUS DISEASES OF CATTLE, SHEEP AND GOATS IN TEXAS. U.S. Dept. Agr., Bur. Anim. Indus., Ann. Rpt. 17 (1900): 356-379.

(16) STOLL, NORMAN R. (1936). OBSERVATIONS ON CATTLE NEMATODE INFFCTIONS, WITH A DEMONSTRATION OF THEIR SECONDARY TRANSMISSION TO GRAZING SHEEP. Jour. Parasitol. 22: 386-407.

(17) ______(1938). TAPEWORM STUDIES VII. VARIATION IN PASTURE INFESTATION WITH M. EXPANSA. Jour. Parasitol., 24: 527-545, illus.

(18) STUNKARD, HORACE W. (1937). THE LIFE CYCLE OF MONIEZIA EXPANSA. Science 86: 312.

(19) SWANSON, L.E., PORTER, D.A. and CONNELLY, J.W. (1940). EFFICACY OF NONCONDITIONAL PHENOTHIAZINE IN REMOVING WORMS FROM ALIMENTARY CANAL OF CATTLE. Amer. Vet. Med. Assoc. Jour. 96: 704-707.

(20) TAYLOR, E.L. (1937). PARASITIC GASTRITIS. THE TRANSFERENCE OF THE CAUSATIVE HELMINTHS FROM SHEEP TO CATTLE. Vet. Jour. 93: 353-355.

Chapter 13

BOVINE GENITAL TRICHOMONIASIS

G. Dikmans[1]

[1] *G. Dikmans is Parasitologist, Zoological Division, Bureau of Animal Industry.*

Only within recent years were the wriggling, micro-organisms known as trichomonads discovered to be a cause of abortion, sterility and breeding difficulties in cattle. Prevention depends on a careful system of management, described in this article.

Bovine Genital Trichomoniasis is a disease of cattle characterized by difficulties in breeding, early abortions, temporary sterility and pyometra (accumulation of pus in the uterus), without an accompanying fever.

The causative organism, technically named *Trichomonas foetus*, was first observed in association with genital disease of cattle by Mazzanti (*5*)[2] in Italy in 1900. He found it in the genital tracts of two cows and one heifer that were slaughtered because of permanent sterility. He considered it to be the cause of the sterility and named it *Trichomonas uterovaginalis vitulae*. The literature contains no further reference to trichomonads in connection with genital disease of cattle

---

[2] Italic numbers in parentheses refer to Literature Cited.

until 1925, when Drescher (*3*) reported finding them in pure culture in a bovine fetus aborted at 7 months. This rather striking 25-year lapse was probably due to the fact that since Bang's discovery in 1897 (*2*) of the organism causing infectious abortion in cattle, the idea that genital disease of cattle manifested by abortion, uterine infection and sterility was Bang's disease or brucellosis, dominated the thinking of veterinarians in this field. Only when breeding troubles occurred in the demonstrated absence of *Brucella abortus* were they attributed to other causes, such as coital exanthema (*9*).

Drescher's report was followed by other reports of similar findings, but they did not settle the problem of the relationship of the trichomonads to genital disease of cattle. Trichomonads had previously been reported from man and various animals. Some investigators considered them harmless, others as organisms responsible for the disease processes in which they were found, while a third group appeared to be of the opinion that trichomonads were secondary invaders unable to initiate pathological conditions but able to aggravate such conditions after they had become established.

Riedmiiller in 1928 (*10*) reported finding trichomonads in nine aborted bovine fetuses. In two of these he found the organism in pure culture, in one he found both trichomonads and *Brucella abortus* and in the remaining six he found trichomonads in association with other bacterial organisms. He described and drew the trichomonad and named it *Trichomonas foetus*.

Experiments conducted by Riedmiiller, Abelein, Witte and Kuest, reported in papers published between 1928 and 1934, showed that:

(1) Trichomonads were found in aborted bovine fetuses, fetal membranes and fetal fluids and in the uterine and vaginal secretions of animals suffering from a condition known as infectious uterine catarrh;

(2) These trichomonads both when mixed with bacterial organisms and in pure cultures were able to produce abortion in experimentally infected guinea pigs and cattle;

(3) Trichomonads occurred in the sheaths of bulls which on clinical and other grounds could be considered as responsible for genital disease of cattle mainfested by abortion, pyometra and sterility;

(4) The trichomonads could be transmitted from male to female and vice versa during coition; and

(5) These manifestations of genital disease occurred in the absence of Bang's disease and coital exanthema.

In carefully controlled experiments Rees and his coworkers (*6, 7, 8*) in the United States were able to infect heifers and further demonstrate the ability of trichomonads to produce delayed conception, pyometra and sterility. A bull was also infected through service with an infected heifer and this bull was subsequently used to infect cows and heifers.

Since 1925 the disease has been reported from several different countries–Germany, France, Italy, the Netherlands, Denmark, Norway, Japan, South Africa, Argentina, Mexico and the United States. The first report of the occurrence of the disease in the United States was made by Emmerson in 1932 (*4*). Since then it has been reported by various authors from different parts of the country.

The protozoan that causes the disease (Fig. 1) is a one-celled microscopic organism with three threadlike whips (flagella) at the front and one at the hind end. An undulating membrane at the back extends almost the entire length of the body. When examined alive, the organism moves across the field of vision of the microscope with an undulating motion; at times it turns and twists and assumes shapes varying from pear-shaped to oval or rounded. The rapidity of its movements depends to some extent on the medium in which it is examined.

Symptoms and Diagnosis

Although *Trichomonas foetus* has been reported as occurring in the vagina of virgin heifers and in the prepuce of a young bull which, so far as known, had never been used for breeding purposes, the usual mode of transmission is by coitus.

As a result of infection one of several things may happen:

(1) The animal may fail to conceive;

(2) Conception may take place and be followed by abortion;

(3) The fetus may die and instead of being expelled may become macerated, while the uterus becomes filled with a characteristic thin, grayish-white, almost odorless fluid; or

(4) A normal gestation and birth may occur in spite of infection.

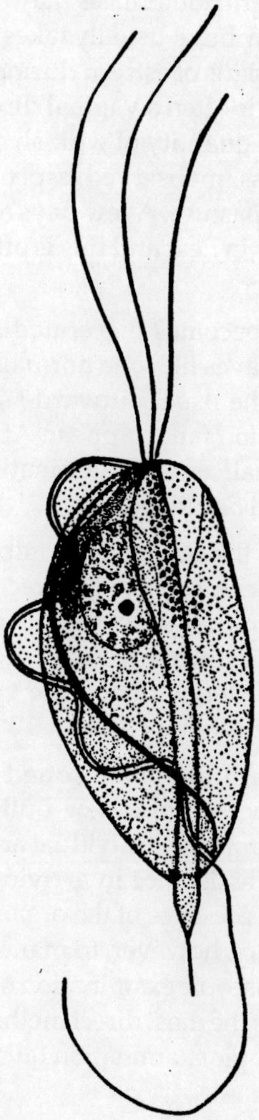

ozoan *Trichomonas foetus*. Greatly magnified.

Animals that fail to conceive may develop a uterine infection manifested by a vaginal discharge. This discharge may be continuous or it may be intermittent, occurring chiefly during estrual periods, which may become irregular.

Abortion due to trichomoniasis may occur at any time during the period of gestation, but it usually takes place 8 to 16 weeks after coition. There are no signs of estrum during this period. A few days before abortion there is often a vaginal discharge. At times instead of a fetus only a small quantity of whitish mucoid fluid is expelled. The abortion may pass unobserved, especially if it occurs at night, in a dark stable or on pasture. A few days after such an abortion the animal usually comes in heat and this is often the first indication of infection.

When the fetus becomes macerated and is not expelled, the animal generally behaves like one normally pregnant. It shows no signs of illness, but the usual outward signs normally indicating approaching parturition fail to appear. At the end of the period of gestation there is no calf and on examination the uterus is found to be filled with the fluid described.

Inflammation of the prepuce accompanied by pus formation and discharge has been reported in recently infected bulls. On examination the preputial mucosa and penis were found to be inflamed and to contain many small nodules similar to those occurring in bulls affected with nodular venereal disease.[3] In bulls the infection usually becomes chronic.

The breeding troubles mentioned very often follow the introduction into the herd of a new bull or new cow; hence the breeding histories of both the individual animals affected and of the herd are of material assistance in arriving at a correct diagnosis. Demonstration of the presence of the organism in vaginal or uterine discharges is necessary, however, to make the diagnosis complete. The immediate microscopic examination of material taken from the vagina or the sheath is the most direct method of making a diagnosis. When direct microscopic examination fails to reveal the organisms,

---

[3] Trichomonads have been reported as occurring in the epididymis and in the ampullae of the vasa deferentia where these enter the urethra; they have also been found in the anterior portion of the urethra.

as it frequently does, culturing the material may prove to be of great assistance.

One method of diagnosing trichomoniasis in the bull consists in the examination, 14 to 21 days after service, of heifers which have been bred for the first time. If trichomoniasis is being transmitted by the bulls under examination, the infection in the heifers will be vaginal at that time and the organisms can usually be readily demonstrated in samples of vaginal secretions. This method has been used with good results in herds having a breeding history indicative of trichomoniasis but in which the presence of trichomonads could not be demonstrated in the older animals. The two principal advantages of the method are that infection can be detected with relative ease and that it can be ascertained with certainty which bull or bulls are infected and transmitting the infection in the herd.

A tentative diagnosis of trichomoniasis can be made on the basis of the breeding history of the herd and of the individual animals. A demonstration of the presence of *Trichomonas foetus* in the suspected animals makes the diagnosis certain. Failure to demonstrate the presence of the organism when the herd history is strongly suggestive of trichomomasis does not mean that the disease is not present; it may simply mean that the examination was not made at the right time and should be repeated.

Treatment, Prevention and Control

There is no specific medicinal treatment for infected animals, and the disease should be handled like any other form of genital infection of cattle.

Cows that abort early in the period of gestation usually recover spontaneously. Such animals should be given a period of sexual rest for about 3 months. Cows showing persistent uterine discharge should be treated for the relief of this symptom. In some cases in which the fetus dies as a result of infection but is not expelled and the uterus becomes filled with fluid, the cervix relaxes when the end of the normal period of gestation approaches and the uterine contents are discharged. In other cases the cervix remains tightly closed and the only practical way of determining the status of the animal is by manual examination through the rectum. In these cases the uterus should be emptied and douched in the usual manner.

Cows that, as a result of trichomonad infection, fail to conceive after repeated services should be given sexual rest until after two or three normal estrual cycles. They should receive such treatment as a veterinarian recommends.

Infected bulls have been considered incurable and their destruction has been advocated as a means of eliminating sources of infection. This advice, while theoretically sound, is not always practical. Abelein (*1*) in 1938 described a treatment that has been used with apparent success in a few cases. It consists in injecting, under spinal anesthesia, 50 to 100 cubic centimeters of a 0.1 per cent solution of trypaflavine into the urethra and rubbing a 0.5 per cent trypaflavine salve into the inner surface of the prepuce. The treatment should be repeated in a week. Washing the penis of bulls infected with trichomonads with a warm 5 per cent oxyquinoline sulfate solution (*11*) once every 8 to 10 days for a period of 3 months has also been reported as a successful method of treatment.

While the medicinal treatment of individual infected animals, whenever such treatment is necessary, is the problem of the attending veterinarian, the prevention of the disease and the handling of a herd into which it has been introduced are largely problems of management. Since the disease is spread principally by coitus, it should be quite apparent that the utmost caution should be exercised in the buying of mature animals as permanent additions to the herd. The breeding histories of all such animals, both male and female and of the herds from which they come should be carefully examined. Bulls with poor breeding records, no matter what their blood lines may be, should not be admitted to the herd except with great caution.

Bringing cows known as hard or difficult breeders on to the premises for breeding purposes may be fraught with danger. It should be determined if possible why the animals are difficult breeders by securing information on the breeding conditions prevailing in the herd from which the animals came.

Permitting cows to be bred away from home may be equally dangerous. An animal may acquire trichomoniasis in the process and later serve as a source of infection in the home herd.

As a rule the disease is well established and a number of animals are infected before the owner or manager becomes aware of it. Since infection is spread by coitus and chronically infected bulls have been considered incurable, a practice followed in certain infected herds is advisable. This consists in restricting the use of infected bulls to cows that either have passed through an attack of the disease or have already been exposed to it. In large herds where a number of bulls are used and there is reason to believe that all of them are infected, the services of each bull can be restricted to certain groups of cows. New, uninfected bulls should be provided for cows that are definitely known not to be infected and to heifers coming of breeding age.

The few cases of trichomoniasis reported in unbred, virgin heifers have occurred in groups of heifers which had been in close contact with infected cows. The presence of trichomonad infection in these heifers is explained on the theory that infection was acquired by contact. There is at the present time no experimental evidence that contact infection can occur, but in order to be on the safe side, it is suggested that the calves and heifers in infected herds be definitely separated from the animals known to be infected.

Recommendations

The precautions that can and should be taken by herd owners and managers to prevent the introduction of trichomoniasis into their herds and to minimize the effects of the disease after it has been introduced may be summarized as follows:

1. No mature animal should be bought as a permanent addition to the herd without a thorough investigation of its breeding record and of the herd from which it comes.
2. No outside animals should be brought on to the premises for breeding purposes without knowledge of their breeding history and that of the herds from which they come.
3. Cows should not be bred outside of the herd and away from the premises without taking similar precautions.
4. If breeding troubles and difficulties occur in the herd, a veterinarian should be consulted. If after examination and consultation it is determined that the trouble is due to trichomoniasis breeding operations should be stopped for a time and available records should be studied in order to determine which animals are infected and which may reasonably be suspected of being infected.

5. The use of bulls known to be or suspected of being infected should be restricted to cows that have undergone an attack of the disease or have previously been exposed to infection.
6. A new bull should be provided for heifers coming to breeding age and for the cows that have not been exposed.

Literature Cited

(1) ABELEIN, R. (1938). BEHANDLUNG VON BULLEN MIT TRICHOMONADEN. Deutsche Tierarztl. Wchnschr. 46: [721]-724, illus.

(2) BANG, B. (1897). THE ETIOLOGY OF EPIZOOTIC ABORTION. Jour. Compar. Path. and Ther. 10: 125-149, illus.

(3) DRESCHER, [L.] (1926). VERWERFEN UND.JUNGTIERSTERBEN BEI SCHAFEN, SCHWEINEN, ZIEGEN. Ber. uber die dritte Jahrestagung der Fachtierazte. Bekampf. Aufzuchtkrankheiten (1925), pp. 190-196.

(4) EMMERSON, M. A. (1932). TRICHOMONIASIS IN CATTLE. A PRELIMINARY REPORT. Amer. Vet. Med. Assoc. Jour. 81: 636-640.

(5) MAZZANTI, E. (1900). DUE OSSERVAZIONE ZOOPARASSITOLOGICHE. OSSERVAZIONE 2a. DI UN NUOVO FLAGELLATO NELLA VITELLA. R. Soc. ed Accad. Vet. Ital. Torino, Gior. 49: 629-631.

(6) REES, CHARLES W. (1937). OBTAINING BACTERIA-FREE PURE LINES OF TRICHOMONAS FOETUS BY MEANS OF MICROISO-LATION. Amer. Jour. Hyg. 26: 283-291.

(7) REES, CHABLES W. (1938). OBSERVATIONS ON BOVINE VENEREAL TRICHOMONIASIS. Vet. Med. 33: 321-334, illus.

(8) REES, CHARLES W. and GARLIOK, GEORGE G. (1939). EXPERIMENTAL TRANSMISSION OF BOVINE VENEREAL TRICHOMONIASIS. Jour. Agr. Res. 59: 769-775.

(9) REISINGER, L. (1928). UNTERSUCHCUNGEN UBER EIN IN OSTERREICH GEHAUFT AUFTRETENDES, JEDOCH NICHT DUBCH DEN BANSCHEN BAZILLUS VERURSACHTES VERWERFEN DER RINDER. Wien. Tierarztl. Monatsschr. 15: [49]-58, 102-111, 169-178.

(10) RIEDMULLER, L. (1928). UEBER DIE MORPHOLOGIE, UEBERTRAGUNGSVERSUCHE UND KLINISCHE BEDEUTUNG DER BEIM SPORADISCHEN ABORTUS DEB RINDES VORKOMMENDEN TRICHOMONADEN. Centbl. f. Bakt. [etc.], Originale I, 108: 103-118, illus.

(11) SCHMIDT, H., TURK, R.D. and SHEPARDSON, C.N. (1937). TRICHOMONAD ABORTION IN CATTLE. Tex. Agr. Expt. Sta. Ann. Rpt. (1937) 50: 14-15.

Chapter 14

CATTLE GRUBS, OR HEEL FLIES

E.W. Laake, F.C. Bishopp, & R.W. Wells[1]

[1] *E.W. Laake is Senior Entomologist, F.C. Bishopp, Assistant Chief and R.W. Wells, Associate Entomologist, Bureau of Entomology and Plant Quarantine*

The annual losses attributed to cattle grubs are estimated conservatively at 50 million dollars a year, but some authorities believe they are twice that high. At any rate, this enemy of beef and dairy producers deserves serious attention. The methods that entomologists have worked out to combat it are described in this article.

Cattle grubs, also called wolves or warbles, are the maggot stage of insects known as heel flies, warble flies or gadflies. Such grubs do a great deal of damage that affects cattlemen, dairymen, packers, tanners and finally, consumers. In the United States there are two species with similar habits. The common cattle grub (*Hypoderma lineatum DeVill.*) has become established in every State, but the northern cattle grub (*Hypoderma bovis DeGeer*) has not yet been found in the South.

Life History of the Cattle Grub

Heel flies (Fig. 1) develop from grubs that have dropped from the backs of cattle. The common heel flies appear during the first

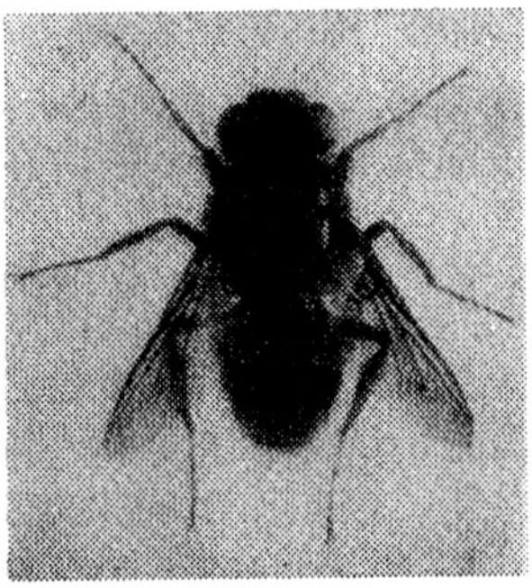

Fig. 1: The common heel fly, female. Enlarged about 2½ times.

warm days of spring and their activity increases as the season advances, until at the end of about 6 weeks the last of them has disappeared.

The eggs, of which one fly often deposits as many as 300, are cemented skilfully to hair close to the skin of the animal, usually low on the legs, particularly just above the hoof (hence the name "heel fly"), but frequently, if the animal is lying down, on the escutcheon and along the hair of the udder and the belly. The eggs of the common cattle grub are usually attached one above another (Fig. 2) and those of the northern species singly. The warmth of the host's body enables the eggs to hatch within 3 to 5 days and the tiny larvae (Fig. 3) emerging from the egg-shells force their way at once through the skin and into the deeper tissues. There the larvae move about constantly but slowly for about 9 months, feeding and growing. They have been found in many locations within the host, particularly in the connective tissue on the surface of the or gans in the abdomen

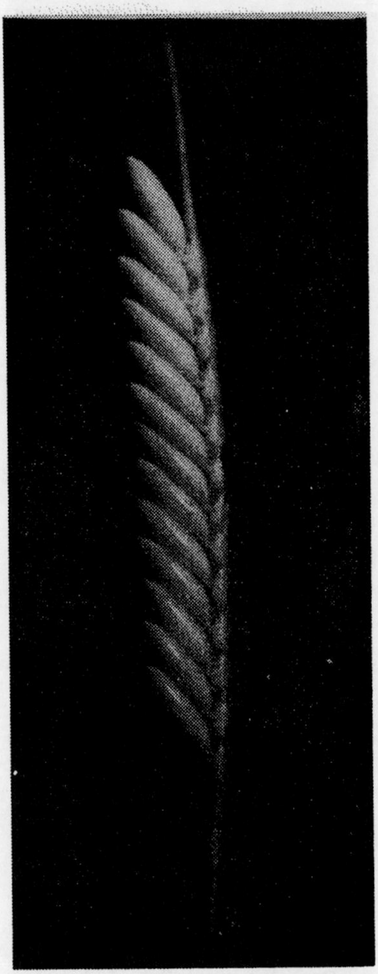

Fig. 2: Eggs of the common heel fly attached to a hair. Greatly enlarged.

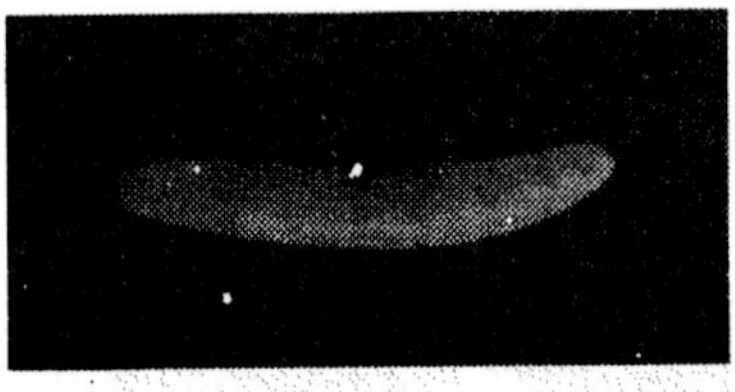

Fig. 3: First-stage larva of the common heel fly. Greatly enlarged.

and between the mucous and muscular layers of the gullet and spinal canal.[2]

The northern heel flies do not appear so early and their activity is extended over a longer period. The grubs of this species are most abundant in the backs of cattle after those of the common heel fly have practically disappeared. Not uncommonly a few of the northern grubs are found in cattle even in August; this overlapping prolongs the fly season in the Northern States and complicates the grub problem there.

The male and female flies live only a few days, rarely longer than a week. They have no need of food and no mouth parts with which to eat. After mating, the females have only one purpose–to deposit their eggs on the hairs of cattle. They do not sting or inflict any pain, as many persons believe. Feeling their touch or sensing their presence, however, cattle are instinctively terrorized.

---

[2] BISHOPP, F.C., LAAKE. E.W., BRUNDRETT, H.M., and WELLS, R.W. THE CATTLE GRUBS OR OX WARBLES, THEIR BIOLOGIES AND SUGGESTIONS FOR CONTROL. U.S. Dept. Agr., Dept. Bul. 1369, 120 pp., illus. 1926.

BISHOPP, F.C., LAAKE, E.W., and WELLS, R.W. CATTLE GRUBS OR HEEL FLIES WITH SUGGESTIONS FOR THEIR CONTROL. U.S. Dept. Agr. Farmers' Bul. 1596, 22 pp., illus. 1936. (Revised.)

After approximately 9 months the larvae arrive at the back of the animal, where each larva makes a hole through the skin (Fig. 4). Shortly thereafter a pocket or cyst, developed from the tissues of the host, forms around the larva and in this the larva remains for 5 weeks or longer. It molts twice after it reaches the back (Figs. 5 & 6). As it grows, it causes a swelling, which usually becomes conspicuous, so that a grubby back has a lumpy appearance. After the second molt the white larva begins to darken, turning yellow, then light brown, then dark brown and finally black when it is about ready to leave the host. Working its way out of the animal's back, it drops to the ground, where it becomes a pupa. If the temperature is not too low, the grubs crawl about for a while before pupating; some go slightly under the surface of the soil, some creep into shallow crevices or underneath leaves or clods, but many have been observed to pupate fully exposed on the surface. In any case, the onset of pupation is not delayed by a search for shelter but begins wherever the larva may be when the temperature is favorable and the process progresses until the fly is ready to emerge from the pupa case (Fig.

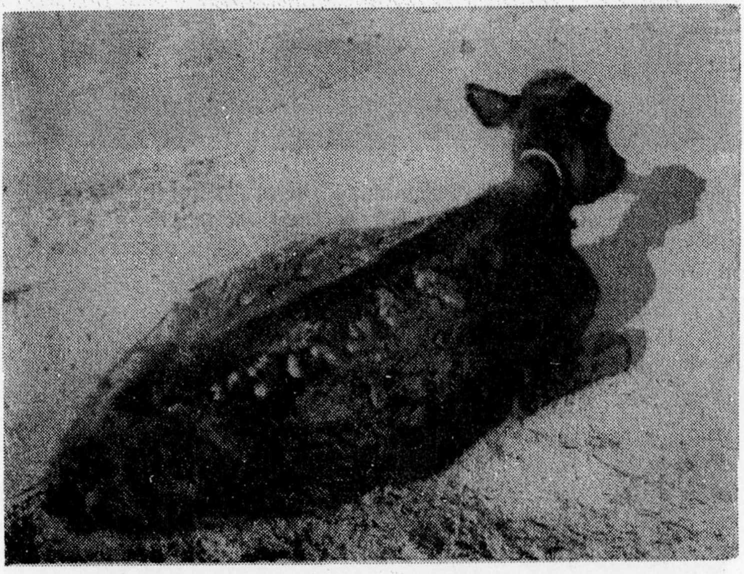

Fig. 4: A cow with holes in its back where grubs are located.

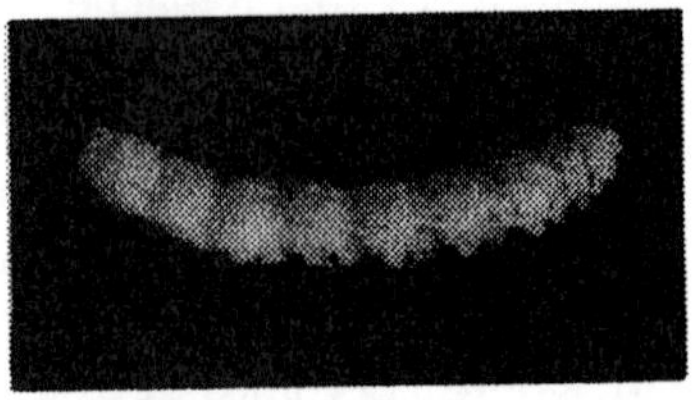

Fig. 5: The second instar (stage between molts) of the grub after the first molt in the back. Much enlarged.

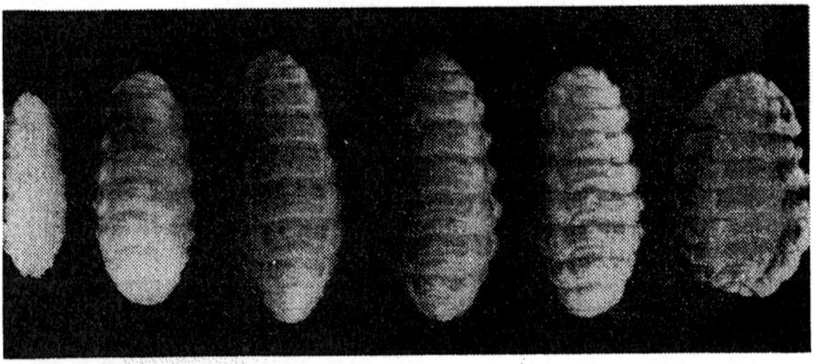

Fig. 6: The third, or final, instar of the grub after the second molt in the back. From left to right, the changes in size and pigmentation as growth proceeds. About natural size.

7). The period of pupation is affected largely by the temperature and varies from 6 to 10 weeks in the natural environment. The shortest pupal period recorded is about 18 days at a constant temperature of 85°F.

Thus the parasite is capable of passing abruptly from a long period within a warm host to a period of comparatively severe exposure on the ground, where metamorphosis takes place and the new generation reaches adulthood.

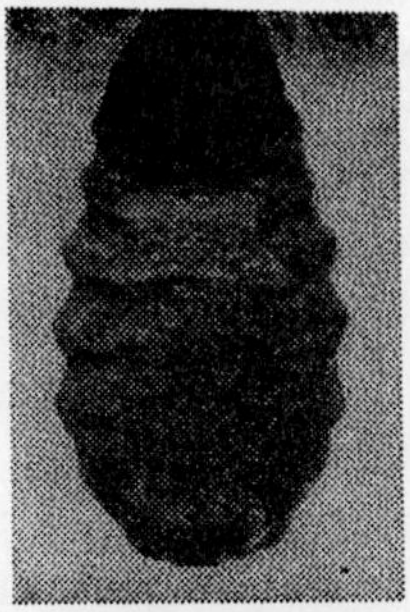

Fig. 7: The pupa case after the fly has emerged. Somewhat enlarged.

Seasonal Occurrence

In the central part of Texas, heel fly activity has been known to begin on the first warm days of February and to extend until the middle of March. Further south it begins somewhat earlier; farther north, later. Thus, if a person started walking at San Antonio, Tex., on February 1 and reached Vermont by the first of August, he might see heel flies active on every warm day along his route. When all grubs have dropped from the backs of cattle at Fort Worth, Tex., they have scarcely begun to appear in the backs of cattle in the northern part of Iowa.

Nature and Amount of Losses

The annual losses attributable to the heel fly and its larvae are estimated to amount to at least 50 million dollars and some investigators put them as high as 100 million dollars. Considering the various ways in which the losses occur, it is evident that the toll is very heavy and that the estimates given are not exaggerated.

The activity of one heel fly is at times sufficient to stampede an entire herd of placid cattle. The fly settles on the hoof or lower leg of one of the herd to deposit an egg; the animal shows apprehension, then fear and finally starts on a mad rush to elude the fly, tail hoisted in a gesture which to all cattle unmistakably means the presence of a heel fly. In the subsequent scramble, the animals may rush over cliffs and through fences. A common refuge is a mudhole or swamp, where frequently many cattle become hopelessly bogged. In addition to incurring immediate casualties, the animals may huddle in shade or stand in water, refusing to feed throughout the day so that they lose or fail to gain weight, as many ranchers can testify. Calves are deprived of milk and the dairyman suffers a heavy loss through decline in milk production, which can be readily estimated. Particularly striking are the losses on large ranches where the cattle are disturbed by heel flies when they are weak from winter conditions and some have baby calves.

Various types of irritation result when the larvae enter the tissues and while they remain. When a large number of grubs are accumulating in the back they cause edema or swelling, often followed by pus formation. Death occasionally follows. The carcasses of cattle slaughtered before the grubs have reached the back exhibit in the affected areas yellowish, watery patches known to butchers as jellied or licked beef. This has to be trimmed away and discarded. Even though the quality of the meat is not affected, the trimming disfigures the carcass and reduces its salability. Another loss to packers is caused by the presence of the young grubs in the gullet or weasand. The grubs have to be trimmed off and many weasands, which otherwise would be used for sausage casings, are punctured and made valueless.

Grubs cause tremendous losses in leather. Commonly as many as 40 and occasionally 100 or more grub holes are found in a hide. Even after the grubs leave the back, the scars remain for several months, impairing the quality of the skin for leather. Records collected by the Institute of American Meat Packers at one plant and its subsidiaries over a 4-year period show that 42 percent of all hides were grubby. According to trade custom, if a hide has as many as 5 grub holes It is classed as grade No. 2 and is subject to a discount of 1 cent a pound. A hide with many grub holes is not considered worth tanning and is sold for by products.

Control Measures

Scientists in many countries have proposed methods for controlling cattle grubs and much attention has been given to the development of effective and practical control methods.

The heel fly is not found in certain areas in the United States–in the Red River Valley of the North, in Minnesota and North Dakota or in the southern part of Florida. Investigators of the Department of Agriculture have concluded that the soils of the Red River Valley are so impervious and the terrain so level that the pupae from grubs dropped from infested cattle brought into this area are kept thoroughly wet while on the ground land thus are killed.

Many substances have been applied to cattle to keep away heel flies and to kill the eggs deposited on the legs of the animals. All have been found to be either ineffective or impractical.

Extensive work on the problem indicates that the best time for attacking the pest is when the grubs are in the backs of the cattle and accessible through the holes they have cut through the skin. Each grub that is permitted to mature and drop to the ground may become a fly and each female fly is capable of laying hundreds of eggs. Squeezing the grubs out with the hands or extracting them with forceps, if carried out systematically on isolated herds, will keep the pests under control. In some areas in closely settled foreign countries, this method is reputed to have eradicated the grubs. Cattlemen in the United States, however, have found it too slow and difficult for general adoption, although some dairymen have practically eliminated the pest from their herds in this way. Among individual animals and breeds there is much variation in the ease with which the grubs can be extracted by hand. They are far more easily removed from animals of the Island breeds than from most others.

Research workers of the Bureau of Entomology and Plant Quarantine have experimented with many substances that can be easily applied to the backs of cattle for killing the grubs before they leave the animals and some have been found to be very effective. The most satisfactory are cube powder and derris powder, the finely ground roots of tropical plants widely used as insecticides. The insecticidal element in these powders, known as rotenone, usually varies in amount from 2 to 6 percent; material containing 5 percent is recommended. When the powder is properly applied, practically every grub is killed and no injury to the animal results. Some of the dead grubs slip out of the back; the others are absorbed by the animal. The powders have been used extensively by dairymen, farmers and ranchers in many parts of the United States; and where they are used systematically, there has been a very marked reduction in the numbers of heel flies and grubs.

The insecticide may be applied dry, by sifting it lightly over the back and rubbing it into the coat of hair with the hands; the process is made easier and the effectiveness of the drug is increased if it is mixed with equal parts by weight of wettable sulfur (325 mesh). Another effective method is to mix the drug in water and apply it thoroughly as a wash with a stiff brush (Fig. 8). The easiest, quickest and most economical method, however, especially for treating a large number of cattle, is to use a power-operated, high-pressure orchard sprayer, controlling the cattle in a chute, as shown in Fig. 9. For this treatment the following formula is recommended:

Cube or derris powder (5 percent rotenone) .... 5 pounds

Wettable sulfur .... 10 pounds

Water .... 100 gallons

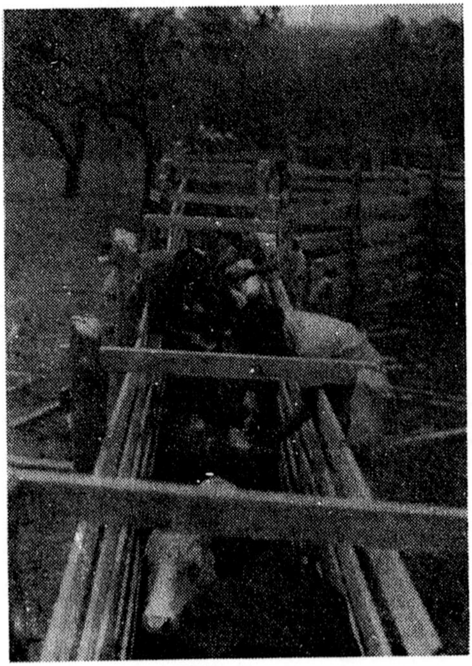

Fig. 8: Applying cube-sulfur wash to the backs of cattle with a brush for the control of cattle grubs.

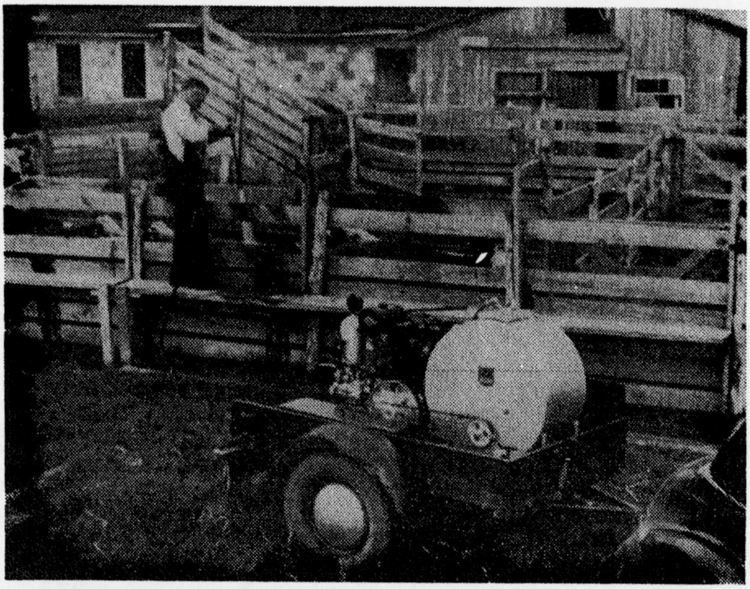

Fig. 9: Cube-sulfur spray being applied to the backs of cattle with a power sprayer for control of cattle grubs

The nozzle is adjusted to produce a medium–fine spray and the operator stands on a walkway beside the chute, high enough up so that he can readily direct the spray downward with force on the back of each animal. By this method a crew of 6 men can handle and treat about 100 cattle an hour, the number depending on the arrangement and convenience of the pens and chute. The spraying method is more economical in quantity of material required than either of the other two.

Detailed information on methods of controlling cattle grubs is presented, in Bureau of Entomology and Plant Quarantine Circular E-496.[3]

[3] WELLS, R.W. THE USE OF DERRIS AND CUBE WASHES IN THE CONTROL OF CATTLE GRUBS. U.S. Bur. Ent. and Plant Quar. Cir. E-496, 5 pp. 1940. [Processed.]

Chapter 15

THE STABLEFLY

F.C. Bishopp & E.W. Laake[1]

[1] *F.C. Bishopp is Assistant Chief and E.W. Laake is senior Entomologist, Bureau of Entomology and Plant Quarantine.*

Most people in temperate climates are familiar with the stablefly or biting housefly, which lives on blood, maddens animals, makes vicious attacks on human beings and can spread some serious diseases. What can be done to get rid of it?

The stablefly (*Stomoxys calcitrans*), also called the stock fly, the biting housefly, and, in the Southeastern States, the dog fly, is found in all the temperate regions of the world. The adults, both male and female, are vicious bloodsuckers with long, piercing mouth parts that on penetrating the skin cause considerable pain to animals or human beings. This fly has been shown to be capable of carrying such livestock diseases as anthrax, swamp fever and surra, as well as infantile paralysis of man.

Although the stablefly is principally an annoyance to man and animals, in large outbreaks it may kill horses and cattle by causing them continuous worry and loss of blood. In some localities–along beaches, for example–it has seriously affected resort interests and lowered the value of real estate by driving people away. It is difficult to control horses when these flies become very numerous; the condition of the animals is impaired, their efficiency is greatly decreased and farm operations are often seriously hampered.

Favorite points of attack by the stablefly are the ears of dogs, hogs and rabbits, which become raw and swollen when numerous punctures are inflicted. The milk production of dairy herds is lowered during every stablefly season, the decrease amounting to as much as 50 percent in seasons when the numbers of flies become large. During such seasons dairy cows and other domestic animals have been known to lose as much as 10 to 15 percent of their weight. The continuous attacks of the flies cause constant fighting and restlessness along the animals and in seeking natural protection they frequently resort to mudholes or swamps, where they may stand for hours, often developing swollen feet and even becoming mired. Such losses and methods of avoiding them have been discussed in a number of publications.[2]

Life History and Habits

The life history of the stablefly is like that of other true flies in that it has four stages–egg, larva, pupa and adult fly.

The eggs (Fig. 1,*A*) are creamy white, elongate oval and about one twenty-fifth of an inch long. The adult females lay the eggs in loose masses or singly on fermenting organic matter such as straw or manure. The flies appear to have a keen sense of smell by which they can quickly detect fermenting vegetation or fresh manure. Usually they crawl into the loose vegetation and deposit their eggs in suitably moist material. The egg hatches in 1 to 3 days, producing a tiny, creamy-white maggot or larva.

Because of careful selection of a breeding place by the parent fly, the larvae have no difficulty in finding ample food nearby. They feed and grow until they are mature, when they are a third to a half inch long (Fig. 1,*B*). During moist warm weather larvae may grow to maturity in 6 or 7 days, but during cool weather this may require a

---

[2] BISHOPP, F.C. THE STABLE FLY (STOMOXYS CALCITRANS L.), AN IMPORTANT LIVE STOCK PEST. Jour. Econ. Ent. 6: 112-127, illus. 1913.

BISHOPP, F.C. THE STABLE FLY: HOW TO PREVENT ITS LOSSES AND ITS ANNOYANCE TO LIVESTOCK. U.S. Dept. Agr. Farmers' Bul. 1097, 23 pp., illus. 1920. (Revised, 1939).

UNITED STATES BUREAU OF ENTOMOLOGY AND PLANT QUARANTINE. STABLE FLIES. U.S. Bur. Ent. and Plant Quar., Insects in Relation to National Defense Cir. 17, 12 pp., illus. 1941. [Processed].

month or more. While developing, they undergo two molts and increase in size but do not change their general appearance. The character and abundance of food, the amount of moisture present and the heat generated by the fermenting vegetation greatly influence the development of the larvae. When mature, they seek a moist, protected place and change to pupae.

The pupa (Fig 1,C) is formed simply by a shortening and thickening of the larva and is transformed directly into the adult fly. The period required for this transformation varies from 5 to 20 days or longer, depending on climatic conditions. Immediately after pupation, the pupa is yellowish or orange in color, but as it ages it darkens, first to light brown and finally to dark brown or almost black.

The fly (Fig. 1,*D*) emerges from the pupal case by splitting open one end and forcing its way out. It then crawls up to the surface of the medium in which the pupa was burled, expands its wings, grooms itself for awhile and takes off on its first flight.

The flies usually feed on blood once a day, but during long, hot summer days may feed twice daily. They also suck moisture from vegetation, manure and fermenting materials. During cold weather they may not feed for several days, but as soon as the weather becomes warm they resume their attacks upon animals.

Laboratory-reared flies begin mating when they are 2 to 3 days old and well-fed females begin laying eggs by the time they are 5 days old. A female usually lays several egg masses, each containing from a few to about 50 eggs. After laying a mass of eggs, the fly must have one to three meals before another mass is developed. Stableflies have been kept alive for a month and a half in laboratory cages and one female under observation laid as many as 600 eggs.

Stableflies are swift, strong fliers. They sometimes follow animals for miles making repeated efforts to bite. That these flies are capable of long flights has been demonstrated by experiments in which large numbers were marked with coloring material and then released. Some of the marked flies were recaptured at distances up to 52 miles from the point of release. It appears from field observations that the flies drift with prevailing winds.

Ordinarily stablefly attacks are confined to the lower parts of an animal's body, particularly the outer sides of the front legs

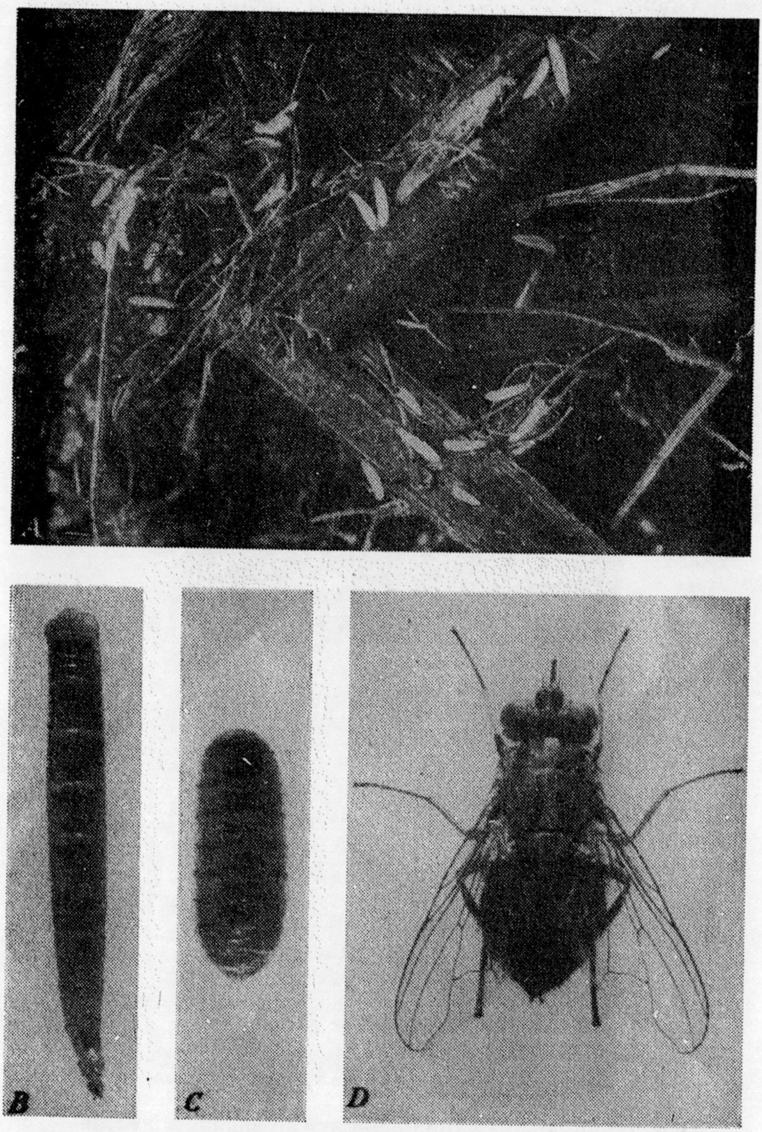

Fig. 1: The stablefly: A: Eggs; B: larva; C: pupa; and D: adult. Greatly enlarged.

(Fig. 2), where the animal's tail is less likely to dislodge them. When the flies are very abundant, however, they may attack all parts of the body. Unmolested flies usually engorge to repletion in 2 to 5 minutes. When full, they rest on a nearby object to digest the meal.

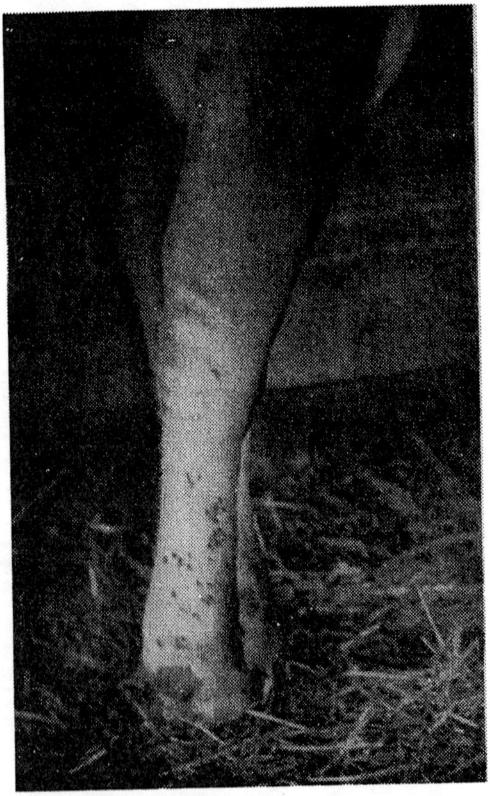

Fig. 2: Stableflies on the forelegs of an animal, a favorite place of attack.

More detailed information on the life history and habits of this pest has been published by Bishopp,[3] Hewitt,[4] and Mitzmain.[5]

Control Measures

The elimination of man made breeding places is of first importance in controlling the stablefly.

In the Grain Belt, straw, especially oat straw, is the chief medium in which flies breed in enormous numbers. The combine has been a blessing in eliminating a considerable amount of this breeding material, but where combines are not used, much straw is still being stacked. Immediate baling of straw that is desired for feeding and bedding purposes is of paramount importance in controlling this fly in the Grain Belt. The stalk butts left after baling should be well scattered. Where baling is impossible, proper stacking of the straw at threshing time so as to prevent the rains from penetrating it will greatly reduce stablefly breeding (Fig. 3).

Manure, especially when mixed with straw, corn husks, silage and alfalfa in barnyards or feed lots, provides a breeding place for many flies. Heaps of grass clippings, celery trimmings or other decaying vegetation in pastures or fields are also fertile breeding places. All this material should be scattered thinly at least once a week or preferably twice, so that it may dry quickly. Neither stableflies nor houseflies can breed in dry vegetable matter and few are able to develop in moist or wet vegetable matter or manure when it is scattered thinly.

In areas where peanuts are grown extensively for the nuts, the litter left in piles after the nuts are harvested has been found by Dove and Simmons[6] to serve as a breeding place for great numbers of

---

[3] See footnote 2, first citation.

[4] HEWITT, C. GORDON. OBSERVATIONS ON THE FEEDING HABITS OF THE STABLE FLY, STOMOXYS CALCITRANS L. Roy. Soc. Canada Trans. (1914), Ser. 3, Sect. IV, 8: 37-42, illus. 1914.

[5] MITZMAIN, M. BRUIN. THE BIONOMICS OF STOMOXYS CALITRANS LINNAEUS; A PRELIMINARY ACCOUNT. Philippine Jour. Sci. (B) 8: 29-48. 1913.

[6] DOVE, W.E. and SIMMONS, S.W. CONTROL OF DOG FLY BREEDING IN PEANUT LITTER. U.S. Bur. Ent. and Plant Quar. Cir. E-542, 4 pp, 1941. [Processed].

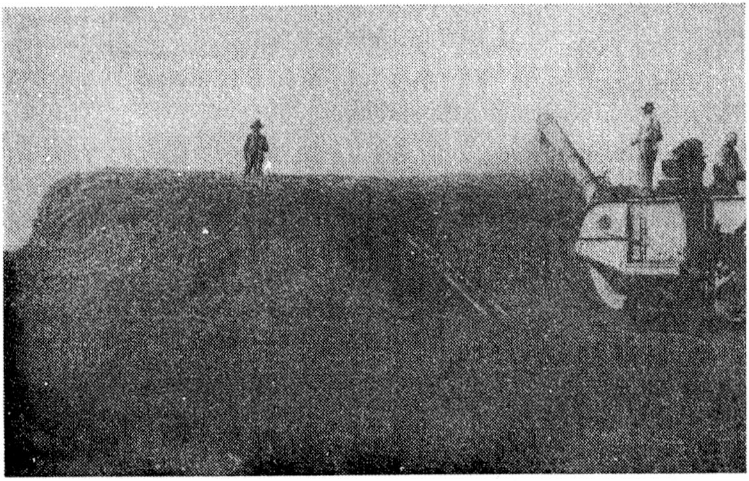

Fig. 3: A strawstack being constructed to prevent breeding cf stablefiies.

stableflies, It is advisable to scatter this litter and plow it under immediately after the peanuts are harvested.

It has also been discovered recently that bay grasses washed up in windrows on certain beaches along the Gulf coast by high tides and storms serve as natural breeding material for stableflIes. Experiments conducted by Simmons and Dove[7] have shown that a mixture of 1 part of creosote oil and 3 parts of No. 2 fuel oil driven deep into the windrows by a power sprayer, using at least 300 pounds pressure, makes such material unsuitable as a breeding place.

Stableflies that develop in natural breeding material beyond man's control can be effectively reduced in numbers by secondary control methods such as traps and sprays. Traps cannot be depended upon, however, for complete control.

---

[7] SIMMONS, S.W., and DOVE, W.E. CONTROL OF DOG FLY BREEDING IN BEACH DEPOSITS OF MARINE GRASSES, U.S. Bur. Ent. and Plant Quar. Clr, E-541, 8. pp. 1941. [Processed.]

The Hodge window trap and electric grids properly installed in barn windows will catch or electrocute most of the flies carried into the barns on animals. It should be remembered, however, that stableflies remain on animals for only relatively short periods while they feed and therefore only those flies that happen to be on an animal when it goes into the barn will be caught.

The cattle fly trap developed by the Bureau of Entomology and Plant Quarantine, which is highly effective in ridding cattle of horn flies, will also catch considerable numbers of stableflies provided cattle go thorough this trap once or twice daily on their way to water, to feed or into the dairy barn; but here again only the flies that happen to be on the animals at the moment they pass through the trap will be caught.

Sprays are undoubtedly the best secondary means for controlling stableflies. Rotenone-oil sprays and pyrethrum-oil sprays properly made not only kill all the flies on an animal at the time of spraying but also leave a residue on the coat which will kill flies attacking the animal within several hours. Rotenone is extracted from the roots of derris and cube plants and pyrethrins from the flowers of pyrethrum plants. Each of these extracts is a powerful insect poison and both are now widely marketed in concentrated form. Five percent of either of the extracts in an odorless, water-white kerosene, also commonly known as a light spray oil, makes an excellent spray. Sprays containing 10 percent of these concentrated extracts in a light spray oil are even more effective, since they afford almost perfect protection for a day or more, instead of only several hours, after spraying. If the animals are sprayed while their hair is dry, rain will not remove much of the toxic residues, since both of these insect poisons are practically insoluble in water. Three-fourths to one and one-half ounces of the spray, depending on the size of the animal, is sufficient for good coverage if it is lightly but uniformly applied with a good atomizer or hand sprayer. Since stableflies bite mostly on the legs and lower parts of the body, it is particularly important that these parts be completely covered by the spray. Sprays are also effective in controlling horn flies and reducing the number of houseflies.

Chapter 16

THE HORN FLY

W.G. Bruce[1]

[1] *W.G. Bruce is Associate Entomologist, Division of Insects Affecting Man and Animals, Bureau of Entomology and Plant Quarantine.*

It can be a serious matter when 4,000 to 10,000 stabbing flies stay on an animal day and night, each taking two meals of blood a day. Here are the facts about a particularly vicious insect and how to combat it.

Probably no fly is more familiar to the cattlemen of the united States than the small black, bloodsucking horn fly (*Haematobia itritans*), also known as the cattle fly, stock fly, cow fly and third-party fly. Throughout the summer months these pestiferous flies congregate by the hundreds, often by the thousands, on the backs, shoulders and bellies of cattle (Fig. 1) and the continuous stabbing by the hundreds of stiletto like mouth parts of the insects causes the animals endless misery. The tormented cattle often refuse to graze during the day and seek protection by hiding in the brush or tall grass until nightfall, when horn flies are less active.

The injury to cattle caused by horn flies is due to irritation and worry, loss of blood, reduced vitality and the production of sores that become infested with screwworms. Like all flies that bite intermittently, the horn fly is also a potential disease carrier.

The interruption to the feeding and rest of cattle interferes with normal digestion and this, together with the loss of blood and the

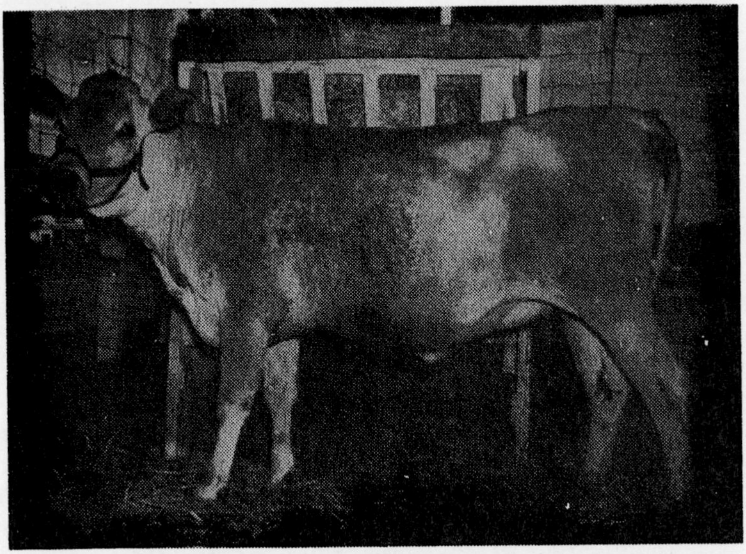

Fig. 1: A heifer heavily infested with horn flies.

expenditure of energy in fighting the flies, results in loss of flesh and reduced milk production.

Horn flies usually feed twice a day, sometimes more frequently. While the loss of blood caused by one fly may appear negligible, the total loss caused by thousands of these pests infesting a herd of cattle may be illustrated by the following example. On a ranch in Texas where there are about 500 head of cattle, the usual horn fly infestation is approximately 4,000 flies to each animal. The loss of blood from this herd is roughly 7 quarts a day or about 2,713 pounds or 312 gallons, a year.

It is difficult to estimate the economic loss due to horn fly attacks, but it is probably not less than 3 million dollars annually. The horn fly may not be the most serious pest attacking cattle, but certainly it is one that inflicts considerable damage and should be controlled.

Description and Habits

The horn fly is about half the size of the common housefly or the common stablefly, but unlike these two larger flies it remains on the cattle throughout the day and night. One peculiar characteristic of the horn fly is its habit of always resting with the head pointed downward.

Horn flies confine their attacks chiefly to cattle, but they are not uncommon on sheep. Occasionally they attack goats, horses, mules, dogs, and, more rarely, human beings. The numbers of horn flies on cattle vary considerably in different localities and at different times of the year. Infestations of 4,000 flies per head are common on cattle in parts of Texas and Oklahoma and frequently as many as 10,000 have been seen on one animal. The most favorable climatic condition for horn fly development is warm, damp, cloudy weather; hot, dry weather or cold weather is unfavorable to the flies. In general it may be stated that temperature determines the presence of horn flies and moisture conditions determine their abundance.

Horn flies leave the cow only to lay eggs. When a cow infested With horn flies voids a dropping, a large number of the flies immediately swarm to it and practically all of them crawl beneath it. Here they lay their shiny brown eggs and within 5 to 10 minutes return to the cow. Protected from the sun and rain, the eggs hatch into tiny white maggots in about 16 hours. These maggots immediately crawl into the dropping, where they feed and grow. Ordinarily they become full-grown in 4 days; then they crawl down into the lower part of the dropping or into the soil to pupate.

In pupating, the maggot draws itself up into a small barrel-shaped object and the outer skill becomes hard and brownish. Inside the hard brown shell the maggot is transformed into a fly. About 6 days after the pupal case is formed, it splits open at one end and a horn flyemerges.

The newly emerged fly is short, leggy, wingless and dark-colored, resembling a small spider more than it does a fly. It crawls rapidly away, seeking a favorable place to complete its development and finally comes to rest somewhere out of the wind, at or near the top of an upright blade of grass or on the side of the dropping. It then starts to distend the abdomen, an operation that requires about 5 minutes. Then follows the unfolding of the wings, slowly at first, until they are about a third unfolded, then quite rapidly. This takes about 2 minutes and is followed by a rather prolonged grooming of the wings with the hind legs. Immediately after the wings are unfolded the body of the fly becomes a light ash-gray color. After 4 or

5 minutes the color begins to darken and 10 minutes later the fly has assumed its final dark-gray color. About 1 hour after the fly emerges from its pupal case it attempts a few short trial flights and then seeks the nearest cow, upon which it settles.

Mating of horn flies has been observed as early as the second day after emergence and fertile eggs were deposited 1 day later. On an average, the change from egg to adult, during the summer months, takes 9 to 12 days. The adult horn fly lives about 7 weeks, during which time a female is capable of producing 375 to 400 eggs.

Control Measures

Fortunately there are several methods by which horn flies can be controlled. The one chosen on a particular farm will depend upon the system of livestock management.

One of the first practical measures is to destroy the maggots in the cattle droppings. This may be accomplished by dragging brush or a spike-tooth harrow over the pasture to break up the droppings or by scattering them with a manure fork or shovel so that they will dry out rapidly and the maggots will not be able to survive. This method of horn fly control is feasible only in small pastures.

The accumulations of cattle manure around barns should be hauled to the fields and spread thinly, preferably by the use of a manure spreader, at least three times a week.

Horn flies are easily killed by most of the livestock sprays now in common use. These sprays are ordinarily made by mixing an extract of pyrethrum with kerosene oil. An economical and efficient spray can be made from any of the various forms of pyrethrum extract sold by reliable dealers by mixing it with the oil according to the directions on the container. Thorough spraying with a good hand or power sprayer, one that will generate a fine mist, is necessary for effective control. In spraying cattle with pyrethrum sprays for horn flies, it is not necessary to direct the spray on to the animal. It is better to generate a fine mist around the animal, especially around the legs and under the belly.

Repellents are often recommended for protecting cattle from horn flies, but they are impractical; it is almost impossible to apply repellents to cattle on the range and the use of these materials, which usually have obnoxious odors and will taint the milk, is not desirable on dairy cows.

An effective cattle fly trap for the control of horn flies has been developed by the Bureau of Entomology and Plant Quarantine.[2] The trap (Fig. 2) is constructed in a gateway of a fence surrounding the water supply or in a lane or other place where cattle will be compelled to pass through it daily on their way to and from water, feed or some frequented place. The framework of the trap is 7 feet wide, 6 feet high and 10 feet long. The passageway through the trap is 33 inches wide and is lined along the sides with heavy, large-mesh wire fencing. On each side of the passageway, set behind the fencing are three trapping elements made of 18-mesh.screen in modified tent-trap construction–that is, the screen on the side of the element facing the passageway is folded in a series of **Z**'s. At the inner fold of each Z is a series of holes through which the flies enter the trapping

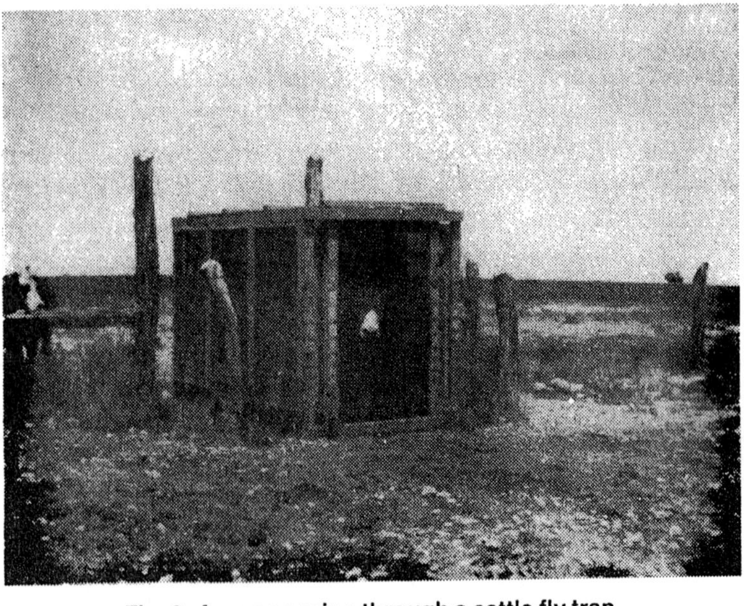

Fig. 2: A cow passing through a cattle fly trap.

---

[2] BRUCE, W.G. A CATTLE FLY TRAP FOR THE CONTROL OF HORN FLIES. U.S. Bur. Ent. and Plant Quar. Cir. E-498, 6 pp., illus. 1940. [Processed].

element. Two sets of curtains and eight weighted strips are used to dislodge the flies from the animals. As an animal passes through the trap, the curtains brush the flies from its back and sides and the weighted strips flap around the legs and belly, dislodging flies not reached by the curtains. The flies attempt to escape through the trapping elements and are captured. The trap is, under many circumstances, the most efficient, economical and practical method of hornfly control.

Some experimental work has been done on the internal medication of cattle for the control of horn fly larvae in the droppings.[3] The idea was to administer by mouth chemicals that would pass out in the droppings and make them poisonous to horn fly larvae. Some of the chemicals proved to be effective, but they can not yet be recommended for general use. Rotenone (all extract of derris, cube and other substances) was the most effective material tested; when administered to cattle daily at the rate of 0.4 gram per 100 pounds of body weight of the animal, it killed all the larvae in the droppings. Zinc oxide, a cheap, common chemical, was also effective when fed dally at the rate of, 1.5 grams per 100 pounds of body weight. Neither rotenone nor zinc oxide had any apparent harmful effect on the cattle.

[3] BRUCE, W.G. THE MEDICATION OF CATTLE FOR THE CONTROL OF HORN FLIES. Kans. Ent. Soc. Jour. 13(2): 41-43. 1940.

Chapter 17

CATTLE LICE

O.G. Babcock and E.C. Cushing[1]

[1] *O.G. Babcock is Associate Entomologist and E.C. Cushing is Principal Entomologist, Division of Insects Affecting Man and Animals, Bureau of Entomology and Plant Quarantine.*

There are four kinds of lice that make the lives of cattle miserable and in severe attacks reduce gains and put the animals off condition. Here these pests are described, together with the best methods for getting rid of them.

Several species of lice prey upon calves and mature cattle throughout the United States. They also attack buffaloes and cattaloes (a hybrid between the buffalo and domestic cattle). The damage they do to animals varies greatly according to the degree of infestation.

In general the number of lice infesting cattle increases slowly during the fall months, then much more rapidly during the winter and spring. Often the animals become literally covered with lice and louse eggs before the louse population begins to decline with the advent of hot weather. This may be true for any one or all the species present. White or light-colored cattle may be so heavily infested as to appear black.

It has been claimed that certain breeds of cattle are more subject to lousiness than others and that Jerseys are the least likely to be infested. Observations indicate, however, that no particular breed is more immune to the attacks of these pests than others.

Heavily infested cattle may in rare cases succumb, but usually the loss takes the form of a reduction of flesh in full-grown animals and slow growth in calves. The mature animals on feed do not make proper gains in weight; they do not eat well and their vitality is greatly lowered. Their generally unthrifty condition is indicated by a depressed attitude and a mangy appearance of the coat and skin brought about partly by constant rubbing, which results in loss of hair in patches, chronic sores and bleeding wounds. During the winter such animals suffer severely. Lousy animals make a poor showing at fairs and stock shows.

Species of Cattle Lice

Four species of lice are known to infest cattle in the United States. Only one, the red louse, *Bovicola bovis* (see Fig. 1), is a biting louse; the others suck blood. The biting louse obtains its food by chewing hairs and particles of skin. It is small and reddish in color when mature, the abdomen having reddish bands running crosswise. These lice, especially in the late spring and often during

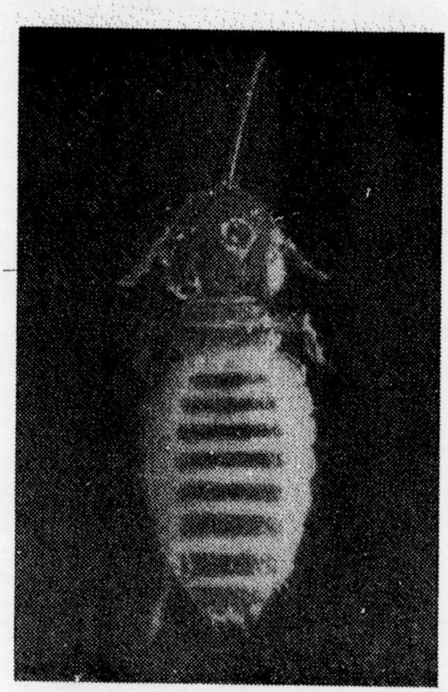

Fig. 1: A biting louse, *Bovicola bovis*, dorsal view.

the summer, will sometimes literally cover an animal and when feed is short on the range calves have been known to die from the effects of such infestations. Young calves infested with the lice are often severely stunted in growth.

Two of the three species of bloodsucking lice that attack cattle are commonly referred to as blue lice. One, *Lingonathus vituli* (Fig. 2), is very common and is disributed throughout the United States. The other, called *Solenopsis capillatus,* is probably more widely distributed than is usually supposed. This louse is a little shorter than the other blue louse but very closely resembles it in general appearance.

These blue or long-nosed, lice develop in patches on different parts of the body and can be very easily seen, especially on the noses of white-faced animals.

Another louse, resembling and related to the hog louse but smaller, is known as the short-nosed or bull-nosed, ox louse (*Haematopinus eurysternus*). The young lice of this species closely resemble the blue lice in general appearance and are often mistaken for them. The young lice usually attach themselves in dense masses or patches on the animal. If not too much disturbed, they remain attached for the purpose of sucking blood until they are sexually

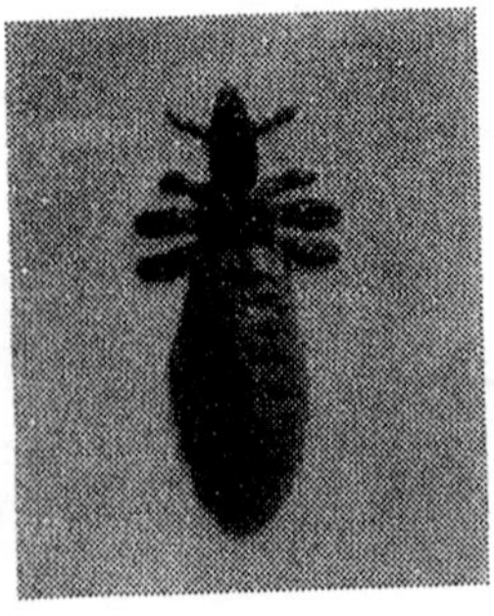

Fig. 2: Long-nosed, or blue, louse (*Linognathus vituli*), dorsal view.

mature, when they crawl about over the animal and reattach themselves to any suitable host that may come in contact with it. This is the usual way in which infestation spreads among cattle. The red and blue lice spread in the same manner, except that they remain attached only for short periods while feeding.

According to Lamson,[2] the eggs of the red louse hatch in 5 to 7 days and the development of the louse to sexual maturity requires 15 to 18 days, whereas the eggs of the common blue louse, *Linognathus vituli*, incubate in 8 to 14 days and the young louse reaches sexual maturity 11 to 18 days later.

In Texas it has been found that a high percentage of the eggs of the short-nosed ox louse normally hatch in 16½ days, though a considerable number require more than 17 days and a few have been found to take as many as 33 days. Imes[3] reports the egg-hatching period as varying from 11 to 18 days, a range that is not surprising, since louse eggs are often exposed to very hot or very cold weather in different parts of the country. After hatching, this louse reaches sexual maturity in 13 to 23 days. The mature female may deposit 30 to 35 eggs during her lifetime.

Control Measures

The remedies suggested for eradicating cattle lice are many and varied, but most of them have very little if any practical merit. No remedy now known can be considered perfect in all respects.

Dipping is the best method of applying insecticides to cattle for the control of lice. For this purpose it is best to provide a well-constructed concrete vat set in the ground (Fig. 3), with suitable chutes and pens for handling the cattle as they are dipped. Such vats are designed primarily for use with large herds or where many small producers can use the same vat. A long vat with straight sides has proved most satisfactory the most desirable type in approximately 26 to 30 feet long, 30 to 36 inches wide and 70 to 80 inches from the water or dip line to the bottom of the vat. This type of vat is also used for dipping cattle to control mange and ticks. For

---

[2] LAMSON. G.H., Jr. CATTLE LICE AND THEIR CONTROL. Conn. (Storrs) Agr. Expt. Sta. Bul. 97. pp. [395]-414, illus. 1918.

[3] IMES, MARION. CATTLE LICE AND HOW TO ERADICATE THEM. U.S. Dept. Agr. Farmers' Bul. 909, 24 PP., illus. 1925. (Revised, 1940).

delousing a few animals. Insecticides in solution may be applied with a bucket pump or other standard sprayer or dry insecticides may be applied with a shaker can and worked into the hair by hand, as described later. Every animal dipped will carry out from a quart to a gallon of dip, depending on its size and the length and condition of its hair.

It is advisable before dipping to see that all projecting nails, splinters and broken boards around chutes and corrals are removed. Other precautions are not to dip any animal while it is overheated and, in cold weather, to do the dipping early enough in the day to allow the animals time to dry before evening. Special care must be taken to avoid heating the animal when arsenic dips are used.

If electric prod poles are to be used in handling the animals, two are generally better than one. Properly handled, these poles are a great advantage, but they should be used only on animals in the

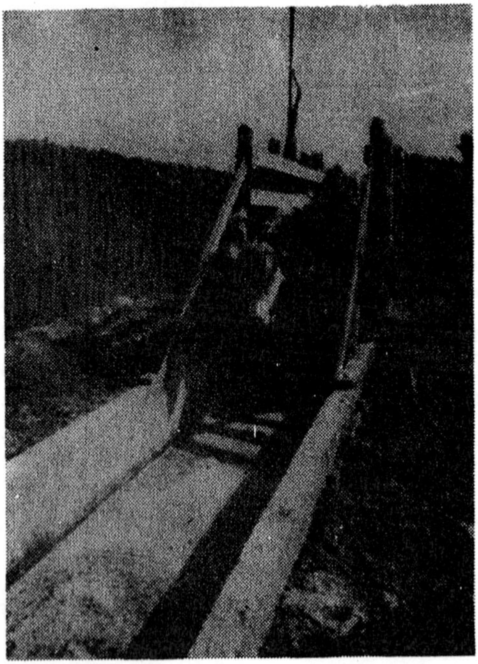

Fig. 3: A dipping vat for cattle, filled to the dip line.

chute; using the poles on animals in the crowding pens may cause them to mill around and become vicious and some of them may jump the corral.

The following dip has so far proved very efficient and safe as well as practical: 325-mesh or finer wettable sulfur, 100 pounds; either cube or derris containing not less than 5 percent of rotenone, 10 pounds; water, 1,000 gallons. The water is put in the vat first and the other ingredients are added to it just before the cattle are dipped. The derris or cube may be put into the water first, then the wettable sulfur; or the cube or derris may be mixed with some of the wettable sulfur in a separate tub, the mixture being added to the water in the vat and the remaining sulfur then put in.

Since the rotenone in derris or cube begins to break down after a few days' use, the dip is good for only 5 or 6 days, after which, if more dipping is to be done a new charge of cube or derris should be put in, but no more sulfur. It is best, however, at the time of the second dipping to clean out the vat and refill it with an entirely fresh mixture.

To insure a satisfactory degree of control, every animal must have its head well ducked at least once during each dipping. The average cattle vat will hold 2,000 to 3,700 gallons of dip, but a capacity of 2,500 gallons seems to be about the most desirable for comparatively small herds.

Owing to the wide variation in the hatching period of louse eggs, it is difficult to arrange a system of dipping that will insure absolute eradication. It has been found, however, that the following dipping schedule is practical and will give a high degree of control:

First dipping–preferably early in the fall.

Second dipping–12 to 14 days later.

Third dipping–17 to 21 days after the first dipping.

Weather conditions will often prevent a third dipping of range cattle at the proper interval. Actual experience has shown that two dippings 17 to 21 days apart will generally give good control. It may not completely eradicate the lice, owing to the fact that on heavily infested animals it is difficult to get every louse wet with the insecticide; again, a few eggs may not hatch until after the second dipping. Louse eggs are not killed by the dip described, nor will arsenical dips kill them.

A number of other insecticidal solutions have been used successfully for cattle louse control, but the sulfur-cube dip is especially effective against the short-nosed ox louse, which is the species most resistant to insecticides.

Coal-tar-creosote dips are effective if used in soft water and at proper strengths.

Nicotine sulfate is also widely used for controlling cattle lice. It is diluted with water in accordance with directions on the container so that the solution contains 0.05 percent nicotine. This dip is very poisonous to livestock and injury may result if it is made stronger than this.

Arsenical dips are widely employed against cattle lice, but neither they nor a dip of elemental sulfur alone with satisfactorily control the short-nosed ox louse. The efficacy of arsenical dips depends on their sodium arsenite content; they should contain 0.18 percent sodium arsenite.

Oil dips are not generally recommended even though they are saponified or mixed with soap.

If only a few animals are to be treated they may be sprayed or dusted with the sulfur and cube mixture. This method is especially desirable for 4-H Club calves or when no vat is available. While one person is working the pump, another can direct the spray and at the same time rub it into the skin. Very low or moderate pressure in the spray pump is better than high pressure, which will make the animal uneasy, nervous and often unruly. In spraying, every part of the animal must be wet, including dew-claws, end of tail, belly and inside of legs.

For the dry treatment–which must be used In cold weather, especially in winter in the Northern States, even if there are a considerable number of animals to be treated–a mixture consisting of 1 pound of either derris or cube containing 5 percent rotenone, plus 9 pounds of 325-mesh wettable or nonwettable sulfur or some of the inert siliceous carriers may be used. The dust-gun method of application has not proved very satisfactory, but hand treatment, although it requires more material and time to apply, is practical and safe. If this method is used, the mixture must be well rubbed into the skin all over the animal. Animals should be treated again in 12 to 14 days and a third time 17 to 21 days after the first treatment.

Chapter 18

CATTLE INJURIES: CAUSED BY INGESTING FOREIGN OBJECTS

L.T. Giltner & John A. Patton[1]

[1] *L.T. Giltner is Senior Veterinarian. Pathological Division. and John A. Patron is Veterinarian, Meat Inspection Division, Bureau of Animal Industry.*

Don't leave your watch where the cow can get it; she may think it is an appetizer. Cattle manage to swallow an amazing number of things that cause serious trouble with their insides.

For some unknown reason, cattle have a tendency to chew and swallow foreign objects. Among those which have been found in their stomachs are pieces of baling wire and barbed wire, bristles from wire brushes, hairpins, hatpins, knitting needles, pocketknives, different kinds of nails including horseshoe and roofing nails, staples and scraps of various kinds of metals with sharp ends or cutting edges (Fig. 1). Besides such objects as these, which are capable of causing considerable damage, other things which probably cause little injury have also been found in bovine stomachs, such as coins, metal tags and badges, watch chains, parts of watches, keys and key chains, buttons, beads, rings, charms and necklaces.

On reaching the first stomach or rumen–more commonly called the paunch–an occasional foreign body may pierce the stomach wall. In most cases, however, the object passes on to the second

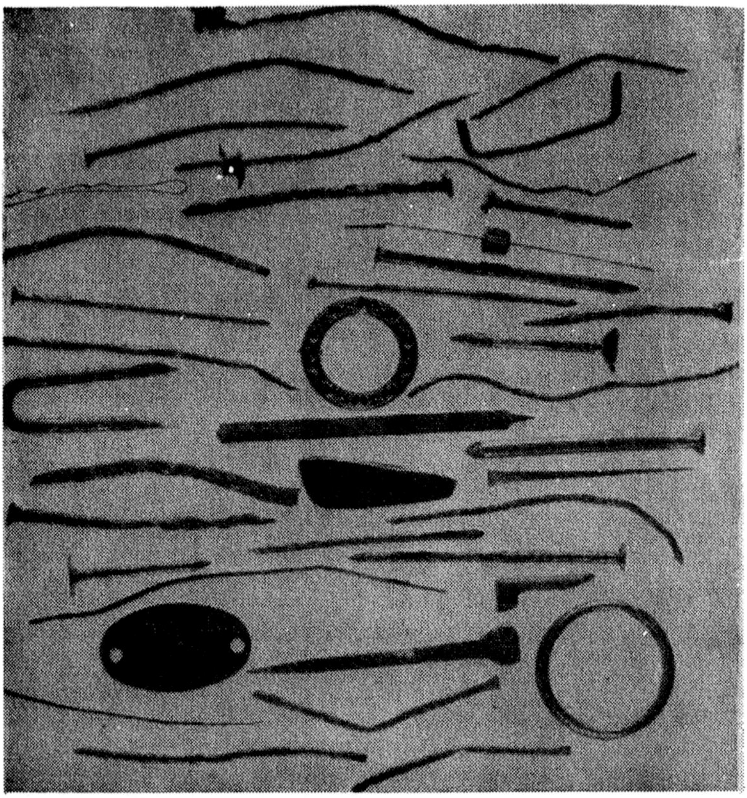

Fig. 1: Metal objects recovered from the stomachs of cattle, include pieces of wire, various kinds of nails, staples, a key ring, a bleeding needle, metal tags, and other miscellaneous articles.

stomach or reticulum, from which it may penetrate the surrounding or related tissues (Fig. 2).

After penetrating the wall of the reticulum, a pointed object may go in one of several directions. In rare cases such an object has been known to work its way through to the external surface of the body. Occasionally it passes toward the liver, causing injury to that organ. The most frequent direction, however, is frontward, toward the heart. This is thought to be due in part to the breathing and chest

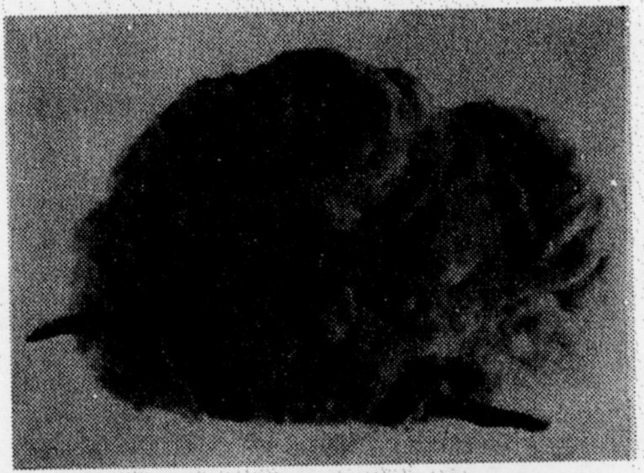

Fig. 2: A portion of a cow's diaphragm which has been penetrated by a piece of wire.

action, together with the muscular contractions of the reticulum. The reticulum lies in close proximity to the pericardium or heart sac, from which it is separated only by the thin diaphragm. After passing through the wall of the reticulum and the diaphragm, the sharp object continues to be forced forward, piercing the heart, sac and may eventually reach and cause injury to the heart itself (Fig. 3). In fact, foreign objects in some instances may even invade the heart cavities.

The condition resulting from penetration of the tissues of the heart region by foreign objects is called traumatic pericarditis, which means injury resulting in extreme inflammatory changes in the pericardium or heart sac and related tissues. Such injuries lead to a train of symptoms and complications which in most cases are extremely serious.

Symptoms

Symptoms are not always readily apparent, as is indicated by the fact that of the cattle condemned on account of pericarditis under Federal meat inspection, fewer than 10 percent of the live animals

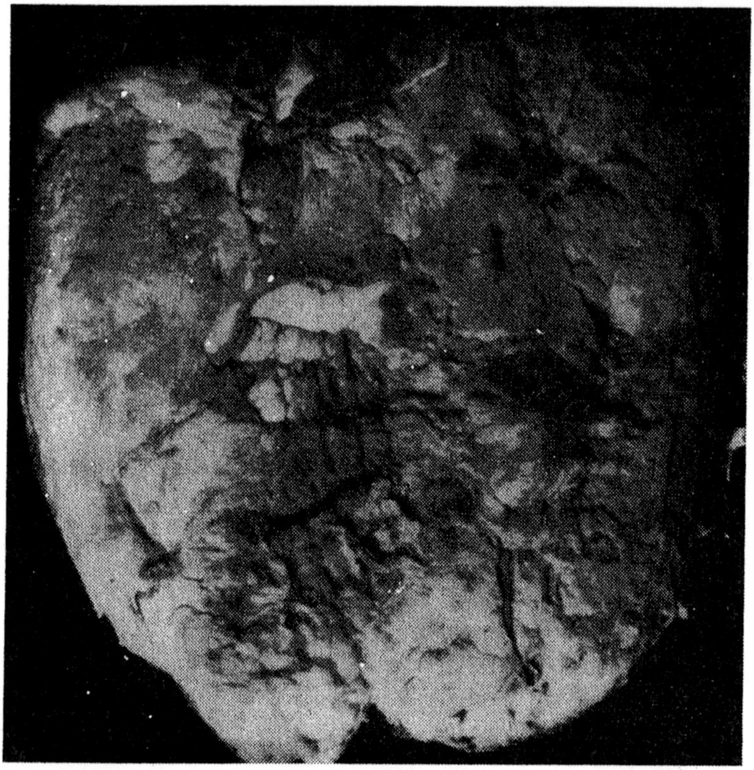

Fig. 3: The heart from a cow with traumatic pericarditis. Note the piece of wire embedded in the heart wall and also the roughened and thickened condition of the myocardium (the muscular part of the wall of the heart) resulting from the chronic inflammatory changes.

shows evidences of the condition, which becomes apparent only on post mortem inspection.

When recognized the symptoms may vary somewhat, depending on the location and extent of the injury resulting from the presence of the foreign object. At first there may be only some evidence of digestive disturbance. In some cases there may be tympanites or distention of the rumen, eructations of gas and indications of colicky pains. The animal may show an anxious expression, avoid motion and keep the back arched. Pain may be evidenced by grunting on sudden motion. The head is stretched forward, elbows spread outward and hind feet drawn under the abdomen. The pulse is rapid and the breathing short, difficult and abdominal in character. There is loss of appetite and little tendency to rumination. In the more advanced cases there are marked frictional heart sounds which may be heard at a distance of several yards and which afford a valuable diagnostic symptom. Frequently there is also a certain amount of liquid around the heart and in these cases a gurgling or splashing sound is heard in addition to the frictional sound. The presence of large amounts of fluid may cause a venous distention, noticeable in the jugular veins, which stand out like cords on the neck and in which wavelike motions may be seen following the heartbeats.

In the later stages, edematous (dropsical) swellings develop on the chest, dewlap and anterior (front) abdominal region. There may be some rise of temperature. As the symptoms increase, respiration becomes more labored and complications such as pneumonia may occur. Diarrhoea is in evidence in some animals. A general loss of condition and emaciation occur. The disease may run a course of several weeks to several months after the first symptoms are observed, but cases of spontaneous recovery are rare. Death may result from direct injury to the heart by the foreign object or from complications resulting from infections.

Treatment

In certain cases, surgical intervention has given very good results and has brought about some spectacular recoveries. The success of surgical treatment depends on the skill of the operator and the proper selection of cases. Some experienced veterinarians have achieved considerable success in diagnosing and selecting suitable cases for removal of the offending foreign body by an operation. Obviously, advanced cases or those in which there is a fever or other evidence of marked poisoning of the system should not be chosen.

Medicinal treatment is of little or no value and when a radical operation cannot be undertaken, it is most economical to slaughter the affected animal as soon as possible after a diagnosis has been made.

Post Mortem Findings

On autopsy the foreign body may be found penetrating the heart wall or free in the accumulated fluid in the pericardial cavity. In some instances the object may pass through the heart wall into a ventricle. Usually the heart sac is much thickened as a result of the inflammatory changes and may in some cases be more or less attached to the heart. Also, as a result of these chronic fibrous changes, the pericardium, diaphragm and reticulum may have firmly adhered to one another. A clear or cloudy fluid exudate or discharge, may be present, but most frequently the heart sac is filled with a creamy pus, due to the invasion of pus-producing bacteria which usually accompany these injuries. The puslike material may have an offensive odor.

Most cases of pericarditis caused by foreign bodies are found on post mortem inspection at slaughtering establishments. In some cases there have been no outward symptoms to indicate the presence of heart lesions or tissue injuries, found after slaughter. Because of the extensive heart lesions, the large amount of pus, the possibility of absorption and the generalized pyemic conditions or distribution of the infection through the body, many of the carcasses so affected are condemned at slaughtering establishments under Federal inspection.

When symptoms of pericarditis are discernible in cattle shipped to market, such animals are sold on a subject-to-slaughter agreement, which means a loss to the owner. Cattle that exhibit no external evidence of the condition but are later condemned become a loss to the packer. Because of the large percentage of condemnation in such cases, traumatic pericarditis is a problem of considerable economic importance. At one station under Federal supervision for example, it accounted for 22 percent of all condemnations for inflammatory it diseases in cattle.

P.B. Becker, of the Florida Agricultural Experiment Station, has reported, in a personal communication, that 59 out of 1,097 dairy bulls on which careful records were kept died from traumatic pericarditis or other traumatisms of stomach, liver, lungs or other organs caused by nails, baling wire or other foreign bodies. In 1940, post mortem examinations conducted by Federal veterinarians on 128,979 cattle slaughtered at one station revealed 6,385 abscessed livers, in 120 (approximately 2 percent) of which pieces of wire or nails were found.

Preventive Measures

Since treatment is of little avail, preventive measures become of extreme importance. Because of the tendency of cattle to pick up various metallic objects, cattle owners, dairymen in particular, should, make a special effort to rid their premises as far as may be practicable of the more common metal objects, particularly baling wire, barbed wire, staples, nails of all kinds and any scraps of tin or other metal that might cause injury if swallowed by animals. It should be possible very largely to prevent traumatic pericarditis in herds by giving thorough and systematic attention to keeping the surroundings free from such objects, particularly around dairies, barns and feed lots.

The importance of paying attention to such details as the careful collecting and safe disposal of all materials that may cause injury when ingested by cattle cannot be stressed too strongly. When repair work is being done about barns, sheds or yards, nails, staples and pieces of barbed-wire or other wire fencing that necessarily become scattered about should be gathered up before the cattle are readmitted. That this pays good dividends is shown by a single example out of many that have come to the attention of the Bureau of Animal Industry. On one large dairy farm under the supervision of a veterinarian, traumatic pericarditis was common and caused the loss of a number of very valuable cattle during a period of about 10 years. After the inauguration of a strict system of surveillance over the "foreign-body enemy" the trouble disappeared and no new cases have since occurred there.

Chapter 19

PAINT POISONING IN CATTLE

L.T. Giltner[1]

[1] L.T. Giltner is Senior Veterinarian, Pathological Division, Bureau of Animal Industry.

Cattle are poisoned by lead paint much more often than most people realize. The author of this article has made a special study of the problem and describes the causes, symptoms, prevention and treatment.

In this discussion, paint poisoning refers to the poisoning that results from the ingestion of any of the lead-containing paints. It is the lead in the paint that causes the trouble.

Cattle may also take into their bodies poisonous quantities of lead from many sources other than paint. Lotions, ointments and salves contain lead and, when applied externally for the treatment of sores, inflammatory conditions and parasitism, may be licked off or the lead may be absorbed through wounds. Lead shot or bullets are sometimes taken up by cattle grazing near shooting ranges; as few as 300 shot have proved fatal to a cow. Herbage in the vicinity of smelters may be covered with a layer of dust containing lead and the forage plants in such areas may take up lead from the soil. The effluent from smelters may contaminate streams with considerable quantities of lead. Dangerous amounts may be deposited on vegetations in orchards sprayed with lead arsenate solution or other solution containing lead; the danger is particularly great if the herbage is grazed before rain has fallen. Old batteries, the exhaust fumes from gasoline engines using tetraethyl lead gasoline and boiled linseed oil are sources of lead to which cattle may at times have access. Soft water conducted through lead pipes and sour feeds such as mashes and milk in leaden containers are sometimes sources of lead poisoning. Finally, mistakes sometimes made in dispensing medicines have caused lead poisoning; for example, sugar of lead (lead acetate) has been mistaken for Glauber's salt or common salt and white lead has been erroheously used for chalk.

Paint, however, is by far the most common source of lead poisoning in cattle. These animals are fond of licking paint, especially fresh paint, from fences, posts, gates, the exterior of barns or the walls, partitions, stanchions and other parts of stables. Also they frequently find discarded paint cans, buckets or other containers and lick enough paint from them to cause fatal poisoning.

Of all the domestic animals, cattle are the most sensitive to lead poisoning in relation to their size, calves being especially susceptible. Frohner[2] states that horses can tolerate 10 times larger quantities of lead than cattle can; he gives the following list of the amounts of sugar of lead that are fatal for certain animals: Cattle, 50 to 100 grams; horses, 500 to 750 grams; sheep and goats, 20 to 25 grams; swine and dogs, 10 to 25 grams.

More farm animals are poisoned by lead than by any of the other metallic poisons and the losses among cattle are greater than the combine losses of all other species. Because of the universal use of paint, the danger of lead poisoning of cattle exists in every farming community. Individual cases in both calves and mature cattle occur frequently and it is not uncommon for a large percentage of a herd to be affected.

Lead acts as a local corrosive irritant to the mucous lining of the stomach and intestines. After being absorbed, it acts on the psychic, motor and vasomotor centers of the brain. (The vasomotor nerves control the dilation and contraction of the blood vessels). Most cases of lead poisoning in cattle are of the acute type resulting from the consumption of large quantities of lead at one time.

The first symptoms are usually marked salivation, slobbering, choking, colic and suppression of the appetite and milk secretion.

---

[2] FROHNER, EUGEN. LEHRBUCH DER TOXIKOLOGIE FUR TIERARZTE. Dritte Auflage, 391 pp. Stuttgart. 1910.

Diarrhoea may occur, but constipation is much more common and bloating often ensues. The symptoms arising from derangement of the central nervous system are most striking and characteristic, although they are often confused with those caused by agencies other than lead. There is a pronounced trembling, accompanied by champing of the jaws, attacks similar to those of epilepsy and a tendency to walk in circles or to push blindly forward into fences or other obstacles. Frequently the affected animals show symptoms of mania, running about wildly with all indications of blindness and colliding with or breaking down objects in their path. Death may occur suddenly during or following such an attack or there may be sleepiness, weakness, paralysis of the hindquarters or other parts of the body and eventually deep coma and death. Animals fatally affected seldom live more than a few days.

Poisoning occasionally occurs in the chronic form as a result of ingestion of small quantities of lead over a long period. In such cases there is a general disturbance of the nutrition of the body, with progressive wasting and general weakness. There may be intermittent attacks of colic, staggering, uncoordinated movements, stiffness of the joints and convulsive seizures. Sometimes there are pustular eruptions in the skin, accompanied by more or less itching. Blindness, wasting of the muscles, ulceration of the mucous membrane of the mouth cavity, abortion and sterility are not uncommon.

In acute cases of lead poisoning, the lining membrane of the stomach and intestines will be found to be reddened and inflamed, with areas of ulceration: The mucous membrane of the intestine has a grayish to black discoloration. The intestines are contracted and the outer surface may be rather pale in color. When the brain cavity or the spinal canal is opened, an excessive amount of fluid pours out and both brain and spinal cord appear congested. Small blood spots are seen frequently on the surface of the heart or under the membrane lining the chest cavity and covering the lungs. In chronic lead poisoning, the body is in a poorly nourished conditions and the internal organs, particularly the kidneys, appear shrunken, owing to growth of connective tissue that has to some extent replaced the softer glandular tissue.

At times the symptoms and post mortem findings do not suffice to establish a diagnosis and laboratory methods must be used. For this purpose not only the stomach contents but also a generous part of the liver should be supplied to the chemist for analysis. Lead is readily absorbed and very slowly excreted from the body, being stored in the liver, central nervous system, pancreas and bones. In cases of true lead poisoning, the recovery of lead from such organs as the liver by chemical analysis is therefore not difficult.

Poisoning by lead from paint or other sources is nearly always the direct result of carelessness or mismanagement. When any painting job is to be done about the farm, cattle should be kept away from the newly painted surfaces and the containers used for mixing the paint as well as the original containers should be carefully disposed of on completion of the work. When the interior of the stable is to be painted, particularly such objects as the stanchions, a nonlead paint that is not poisonous should be used; in general, a good whitewash is quite satisfactory for large wall areas. Before new paint is applied, the surfaces should be scraped to remove old paint scales, which should be safely disposed of.

The animals should not be allowed access to any other sources of lead such as those mentioned at the beginning of this article. Since treatment is usually not very satisfactory, preventive measures are particularly important and should be kept in mind by the stock owner.

The medicinal treatment of lead poisoning is to a large extent symptomatic. When an animal is in a state of great excitement, the veterinarian usually administers such hypnotics or anticonvulsants as chloral hydrate. After the animal has become paralyzed, such agents should not be employed. One of the commonest antidotes is Epsom salts, in a purgative dose; these salts bring about a precipitation of the lead in the form of an insoluble lead compound and tend to prevent further absorption. In recent years veterinarians have obtained some favorable responses through the intravenous injection of calcium gluconate.

Chapter 20

NUTRITIONAL DISEASES OF CATTLE

Louise L. Madsen[1]

[1] *Louis L. Madsen is Nutritionist, Animal Nutrition Division, Bureau of Animal Industry.*

A discussion of the symptoms, causes, prevention and treatment of disorders due to mineral deficiencies, vitamin deficiencies and certain other conditions associated with nutrition in cattle.

Faulty nutrition is often responsible, directly or indirectly, for large economic losses in the cattle industry. Recognition of this has stimulated research in this field and much is being accomplished.

It is becoming evident that the so-called nutritional diseases that occur under practical conditions on the farm or range are not always fatal. Undoubtedly, greater losses result from decrease in rate of growth and economy of production, reproductive failures and increased susceptibility to certain infectious and parasitic diseases than from death. The vital role of nutrition in maintaining health in cattle and other farm animals has been recognized for many years and this accounts for the careful attention given by livestock producers and veterinarians to providing an adequate diet as a part of the programme for the treatment or prevention of many diseases.

In feeding studies much attention is given to comparing the rate of gain or the economy of production of milk or butterfat in animals fed certain feeds or feed combinations. Extensive tables of feed values are being compiled and it is becoming increasingly evident that the value of a feed for any given purpose depends on its content of essential nutrients, which can now be determined to a large extent by chemical analysis. With this knowledge at hand it is possible to supplement deficient rations with the necessary essential nutrients–minerals, vitamins or protein–and obtain good results with feeds which, when fed alone, have a relatively low value or even cause nutritional diseases. Knowledge of the essential nutrients has also led to improved methods of growing, harvesting, storing and processing feeds in order to increase or preserve nutritive values. Recognition of these facts has often made it possible for a thriving cattle industry to be built up in sections where cattle feeding for either dairy or beef purposes was not entirely successful because of some rather obscure factors that limited the growth or production or affected the health of the animals.

Some nutritional diseases are due to a deficiency of essential nutrients and others to overfeeding or dietary imbalance or the presence of toxic substances in the feed. Characteristic symptoms of many nutritional diseases of cattle are now well established and by study and observation livestock men and others concerned can learn to recognize these conditions and overcome them before serious losses result. Prevention, however, is the most successful means of control.

Before the common nutritional diseases are considered, it is important to emphasize that in many cases the results obtained in overcoming them have been so dramatic that some minerals and vitamins have come to be popularly regarded as almost in the nature of stimulating drugs or medicines. This is a mistaken point of view and has often led to unnecessary expense and disappointment when more of the essential factors are added to an already adequate ration. Results from increasing the intake of essential substances are obtained only when the ration is deficient in them. Further- more, when a ration is deficient in several essential nutrients, all of them must be supplied for optimum results.

The Mineral-Deficiency Diseases

The minerals which have received the most attention in cattle-nutrition studies are phosphorus, calcium, magnesium, sodium and chlorine, iodine, iron, copper and cobalt. Other minerals such as fluorine and selenium have been investigated largely from the standpoint of their toxicity. The mineral-deficiency diseases and the conditions caused by toxic minerals usually produce fairly typical symptoms and gross alterations in the body tissues. Blood and tissue analyses as well as microscopic examination of tissues are further aids to diagnosis.

Calcium and Phosphorus Deficiency

The first symptom usually noted in cattle receiving too little phosphorus or calcium is a depraved appetite (pica), particularly evident in phosphorus deficiency (*51*).[2] Phosphorus-deficient cattle frequently chew and eat bones (osteophagia) or other material such as wood, hair, putrid flesh, soil, rocks, leather, feathers, ere., in an effort to get additional phosphorus (Fig. 1). Consumption of putrid bones, flesh and other carcass material may lead to toxic symptoms and death from botulism if the material is infected with *Clostridium botulinum*, as is often the case. Loin disease of cattle in Texas and lamsiekte of sheep and cattle in South Africa are caused by toxin obtained in putrid material consumed in an effort to satisfy the craving for phosphorus. As the deficiency progresses, there are marked loss of appetite, emaciation, lowered efficiency of food utilization, weak bones, stiff joints (creeps), decreased milk flow, failure to come in heat normally, small calf crop and a generally unthrifty appearance.

When laboratory facilities are available, phosphorus deficiency can be diagnosed either by analyzing the forage accessible to the cattle or by blood analysis for phosphorus. A large decrease in total inorganic phosphorus in the blood is the first indication of phosphorus deficiency.

Calcium deficiency in cattle, including lactating dairy cows, is very rare, especially when the animals are fed rations containing liberal amounts of roughage. Isolated cases of calcium deficiency may occur, however, under unusual feeding conditions. Becker, Neal and Shealy (*9*) report that dairy cows on low calcium rations

[2] Italic numbers in parenthesis refer to Literature Cited.

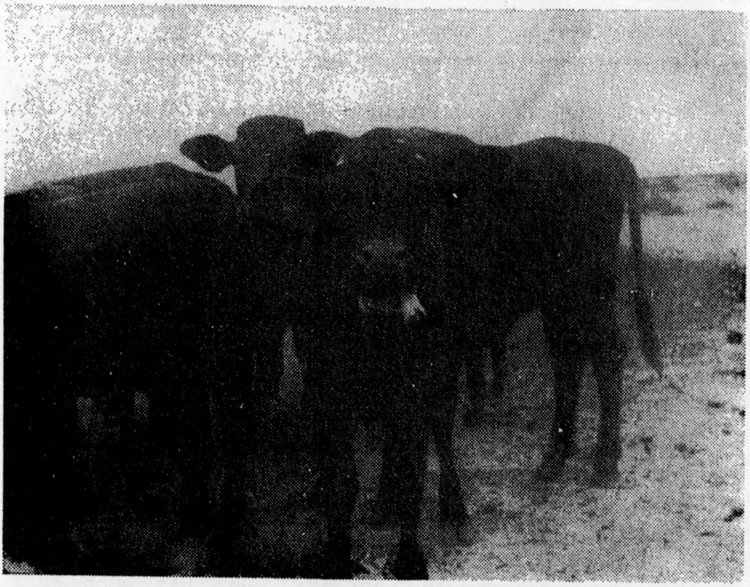

Fig. 1: Phosphorus-deficient cattle often chew bones and other nonfood material in an effort to remedy the deficiency.

frequently suffered bone fractures and gave less milk than when adequate calcium supplements were fed. The calcium-deficient cows remained in good condition, however and did not show lethargy and stiffness, which is characteristic of advanced phosphorus deficiency. Adult cattle usually show only a slight decrease in blood calcium when they are on calcium-deficient rations; younger animals show a greater decrease, but it is practically never as great as the decrease in blood phosphorus in phosphorus deficiency.

An inadequate phosphorus or calcium intake over a long period leads to a gradual decrease in the body reserves of these elements. The largest reserve of calcium and phosphorus is in the bones and if abnormal demands are made on this storage depot to meet the requirements of the body, the deficiency symptoms described may gradually develop. In general, during periods of rapid growth and heavy lactation cattle use more calcium and phosphorus than at any other time. Dairy cows frequently secrete more calcium and phosphorus. in their milk during periods of heavy lactation than is obtained from the feed consumed. The extra calcium and phosphorus come from the bones. Any deficit is usually made good later when the milk flow declines or during the succeeding dry period.

Phosphorus deficiency is much more common in cattle than calcium deficiency. Cattle grazing in range areas or on farm pastures may develop phosphorus deficiency during periods of drought, especially in regions where the available soil phosphorus is rather low. When the feed supply is restricted owing to drought, overgrazing or other causes, there may be a phosphorus shortage that would not ordinarily develop if ample forage was available.

In some sections of the country many dairy and beef cattle are fed primarily on roughage, such as alfalfa, with little or no grain to supplement it. Alfalfa is not usually rich enough in phosphorus to be depended upon as the sole source of this mineral, particularly if it is grown under conditions of relatively low soil fertility and low soil moisture. Most hays are even lower in phosphorus than alfalfa. In sugar-beet-producing areas, beet pulp is fed in addition to hay. Any beet by product is very low in phosphorus, as is corn silage; so a combination of either one with hay is apt to lead to a deficiency of this mineral. Wintering animals in stubble fields with free access only to cereal straw, corn fodder, prairie hay or other similar low-phosphorus feeds may also lead to phosphorus deficiency unless some cereal grains, protein concentrates or phosphorus-rich mineral mixture is supplied. Pregnant and lactating cows or young growing animals are more susceptible to phosphorus deficiency than mature stock cattle.

Prevention and Treatment

Calcium and phosphorus deficiency can usually be avoided or overcome by giving animals an adequate supply of these minerals through the use of feeds that are good sources, the feeding of calcium- and phosphorus-rich mineral supplements or increasing the mineral content and yield of available forage by fertilizing the soil on which the crops are grown.

Investigations of the Bureau of Animal Industry in cooperation with the Texas Agricultural Experiment Station and the King Ranch in south Texas have shown that many cattle in the Gulf coast area graze in phosphorus-deficient or semi-phosphorus-deficient ranges.

Preliminary results obtained in these experiments by hand-feeding a mineral mixture rich in phosphorus to beef cattle on phosphorus-deficient range are given in Table 1. The phosphorus supplements consisted of bonemeal and disodium phosphate. They were fed individually so as to supply the dry cows with 6.5 grams of phosphorus and the lactating cows with 14.3 grams of phosphorus per head daily, in addition to that received from range forage. It is obvious from the data that feeding a phosphorus supplement costing $2.60 per cow per year raised the calf crop considerably, improved the growth rate of calves and increased the value of the calves at weaning time by an average of $10.44 and that of the yearling heifers by an average of $12.19. It is obvious also that adequate feeding of existing herds is a rapid and economical means of increasing beef production.

Table 1: Preliminary comparisons of gains and other production data on cows and calves fed a phosphorus supplement and on similar cattle receiving only range vegetation[1].

Item	*Cattle fed phosphorus supplement in addition to the range forage*	*Cattle on range fed no additional phosphorus*
Calf crop (2-year average) .... percent	83	58
Cows producing calves for 2 consecutive years .... do	72	21
Average weaning weight of calves .... pounds	499	421
Average weaning weight of calves prorated to all cows .... do	448	320
Value of calf at weaning time[2] .... dollars	39.92	29.48
Weight of heifers at 1 year of age .... pounds	541	441
Value of yearling heifers less cost of supplement fed from weaning to 1 year[2] .... dollars	43.06	30.87
Annual cost of phosphorus supplement per cow .... do	2.60	———

[1] Data obtained by Bureau of Animal Industry, Texas Agricultural Experiment Station and the King Ranch, Kingsville, Tex., cooperating.

[2] Calves from cows fed phosphorus supplement were valued at 8 cents a pound and those from the cows that received no additional phosphorus were valued at 7 cents a pound.

Under practical range conditions, phosphorus supplements are usually fed free choice. Soluble phosphorus salts such as disodium phosphate, may be given in the drinking water if the source of water can be controlled. The experience of H. Welch, of the Montana Agricultural Experiment Station, in supplying range cattle with phosphorus supplements indicates some of the problems involved. He writes:[3]

We have been using bonemeal and other phosphorus-containing supplements for approximately 20 years in the Montana phosphate-deficient areas. Feeding bonemeal without salt has 2 principal drawbacks. One is that when put out in a box for range cattle, it blows out badly in windy areas: salt helps to bind it together and prevents this blowing. Second, in any bunch of bone-chewing cattle there are several individuals that refuse to eat bonemeal at all unless mixed with salt. Another objection to pure bonemeal is that after it becomes damp the flies will soon deposit eggs and the bonemeal will become a mass of fly larvae. However, some cattlemen do use the bonemeal in separate compartments of the salt box.

Extensive experiments with disodium phosphate, either straight or mixed with salt, in our hands, have not been as satisfactory as with bonemeal. As far as we can tell, the disodium phosphate is tasteless, but the cattle almost universally found it unpalatable. The same was true of monocalcium phosphate, of phosphate rock origin, containing up to 45 percent P_2O_5, which proved entirely unpalatable to cattle on account of its acid taste.

I mention all these things because it seems to the casual observer that an existing condition of aphosphorosis [phosphorus deficiency] can be remedied by the use of bonemeal and that is all there is to it. In actual fact, however, there are some difficulties in entirely remedying the situation, because of the difficulties encountered in getting an adequate dose of the supplement into the cattle.

Mineral mixtures fed on the range or in farm pastures should be placed in well-constructed boxes that protect the contents as much as possible from blowing out or being wet. A satisfactory mineral box is shown in a recent publication from the Florida Agricultural Experiment Station (*48*).

---

[3] Communication to the Animal Nutrition Division, Bureau of Animal Industry.

The phosphorus requirement of lactating dairy cows needs special attention, particularly in areas where there is a deficiency of this mineral in the soil and consequently a low content in the pasture grass and harvested forage. If the cows are fed a liberal amount of grain, including a protein-rich concentrate such as wheat bran, cottonseed, linseed or soybean meal and a roughage, their phosphorus and calcium intake is usually adequate. For very heavily producing dairy cows, a mineral mixture of bonemeal and salt or some other calcium-phosphorus supplement may be added to the grain mixture at the rate of 1 to 2 percent when necessary. There is little experimental evidence indicating that increased amounts of calcium in the form of mineral supplements have proved beneficial for either growing or lactating cattle when the animals were receiving liberal quantities of feeds of normal composition.

Lactating animals fed roughage with little or no grain should have access to a mineral mixture such as bonemeal alone or 2 parts of bonemeal to 1 of common salt, according to the appetites of the animals, in order to insure an adequate phosphorus intake. Ground rock phosphate, either raw or as a superphosphate, is likely to contain too much fluorine and arsenic and should not be used in livestock feeding. Purified phosphate salts are available. Dicalcium phosphate and disodium phosphate are probably the most widely used forms of phosphate salts, but they have often proved to be rather unpalatable to cattle and are therefore most successfully used mixed with salt or as a constituent of a grain mixture. Bonemeal and the other calcium-containing salts mentioned also provide an abundance of calcium and when these supplements are used it is not necessary to add additional calcium in the form of calcium carbonate. If a ration needs the addition of calcium only, a good grade of ground calcium carbonate or oystershell is usually the cheapest source of this mineral.

Phosphorus Deficiency and Parturient Hemoglobinemia of Dairy Cows

Madsen and Nielsen (*25, 26*) have described a disease of high-producing dairy cows which most frequently occurs 2 to 3 weeks after the birth of the third to the sixth calf and is characterized by anemia (decrease of red blood cells), hemoglobinemia (hemoglobin or red blood pigment in solution in the serum), hemoglobinuria (hemoglobin in the urine) and general weakness. The disease is common in the intermountain areas of the United. States and has been reported from Norway, Sweden, Denmark, Finland, Austria, Ireland and Scotland. It may be confused with other conditions causing hemoglobinuria.

Madsen and Nielsen show a definite relationship between the occurrence of the disease and the ration fed. The disease is most common during the winter, especially when the cows are fed on alfalfa and sugar-beet pulp. No cases have been observed in beef cows. Other characteristic symptoms are loss of appetite, decrease in milk production, rapid pulse, cold and blanched teats, drooping ears, gaunt appearance, weakness, staggering gait, constipation or diarrhoea, depraved appetite, increased water consumption, an odor of acetone on the breath, and, in some cases, milk tinted with hemoglobin. Cows that do not die of the disease usually start to recover after the fifth day of illness and there is partial or complete recovery in a period varying between a week and several months. Cows fed liberal amounts of grain usually recover faster than those kept on their original ration of alfalfa and beet pulp.

The principal blood findings in this disease are a marked reduction in red blood cells and a very marked drop in inorganic phosphorus content. As already noted, the blood plasma is often tinged with hemoglobin. Treatment consisting of intravenous injection of dibasic sodium phosphate followed by drenches with the same material or with bonemeal have been quite successful. No cases have been observed by these authors where cows were liberally fed with gram during the lactation period. Regular feeding of a mineral supplement such as bonemeal is also indicated, particularly with low-phosphorous feeds such as beet pulp.

Magnesium Deficiency in Calves

When young calves are fed on milk without forage or a grain supplement for more than a few weeks, they invariably develop a severe disorder characterized by irritability, nervousness and loss of appetite. In later stages the animals have convulsions. Duncan and associates (*14*) in describing this symptom state:

The animal, apparently temporarily blinded, will run into obstacles or becoming confused will turn in circles until its balance is completely destroyed. As the convulsions become more violent, the calf may fall on its side with the legs rigid and alternately extended and contracted; there is frothing at the mouth and profuse salivation. These attacks may last continuously for several minutes or, intermittently, for a longer time. Young calves seem to be able to withstand several such convulsions but older calves usually succumb to the first attack.

Such symptoms are associated with low blood magnesium. Moore and coworkers (*31*), in connection with the Michigan work on magnesium have described the lesions (tissue changes) in calves fed rations low in magnesium. The principal findings were calcification of the yellow elastic fibers of the endocardium (membrane lining the interior of the heart), in the walls of the larger veins and arteries, on the surface of the diaphragm and in the trabeculae (fibrous bands extending into the interior) and capsule of the spleen. Degeneration and calcification were also found in the Purkinje system (conducting fibers) of the heart. Kidney and liver damage was also found in some cases. These workers suggest a possible relationship between diets low in magnesium and arteriosclerosis of human beings. (Typical blood-vessel lesions found in calves suffering from magnesium deficiency are shown in Fig. 2).

Ordinary diets of forage and grains contain enough magnesium that disorders due to magnesium deficiency are not likely to occur in calves under practical conditions unless they are fed too long on milk without access to supplementary feeds. Feeds rich in magnesium are legume and grass hays, cottonseed, linseed and soybean meal, wheat bran, wheat middlings, beet pulp and hominy feed. Huffman and Duncan (22) report that 15 to 20 milligrams of magnesium as magnesium carbonate ($MgCO_8$) or magnesium oxide (MgO) per pound of body weight maintained plasma magnesium values and prevented the manifestations of magnesium deficiency. Under the same conditions 8 to 10 milligrams of magnesium from natural feeds per pound of body weight was equally effective, indicating that the magnesium of natural feeds is more readily utilized by calves.

Grass Tetany

Grass tetany is a highly fatal disease of cattle characterized biochemically by lowered blood magnesium and calcium. It occurs most often within 2 weeks after the animals have been turned out to good pasture. The disease has received more attention in Holland, Great Britain and New Zealand than elsewhere, although it is known to occur also in the United States (*28, 45*).

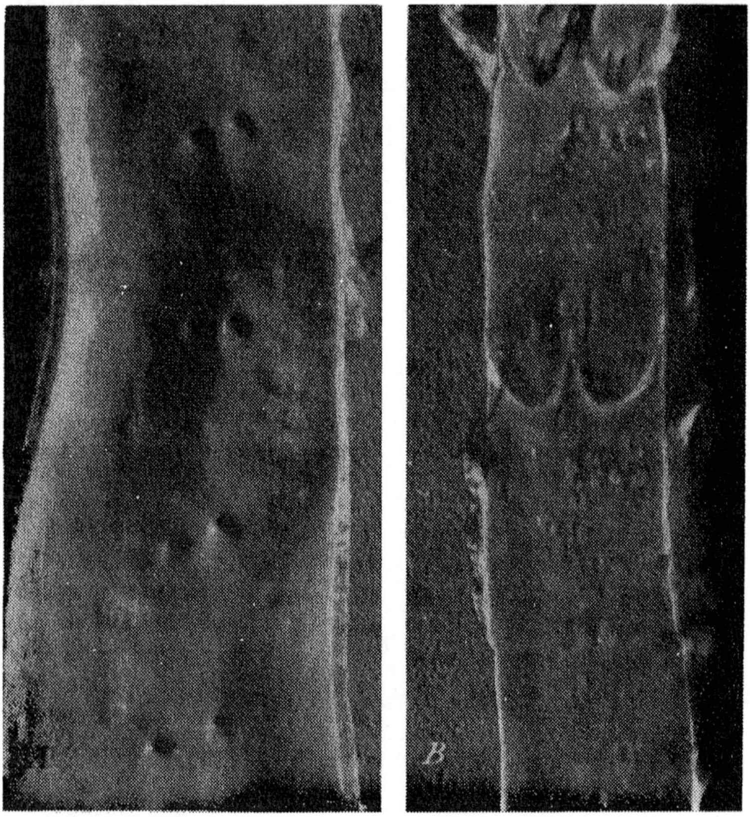

Fig.2: Calves suffering from magnesium deficiency frequently have calcification of the blood vessels: *A*: Calcification of the aorta; *B*: calcification of the jugular vein. (Courtesy of Michigan Agricultural Experiment Station).

Sjollema (*49*) describes this condition vividly:

Usually the initial signs are nervousness, restlessness, grazing apart from the herd, lack of appetite, muscle-twitching, unsteady gait, spreading of the hind limbs, gnashing of the teeth, rolling of the eyes, an anxious or wild look resulting from abnormal eye muscle contraction, frothing at the mouth and abundant salivation. Some animals low continuously. The ears stand erect and certain muscles, *e.g.* those of the tall, are in tetanic contraction. Abnormal contraction of the neck muscles causes a backward thrust of the head and similar contraction of the masticatory muscles results in trismus [lockjaw]. . . clonic-tonic convulsions [alternate rigidity and relaxation] appear and the animal strikes heavily with all four limbs. During these cramps the animal is in a state of intense excitement and alternately falls down and gets up with a jerk, the attempt to rise being often unsuccessful. The animals also run against walls, into ditches, etc., violent cramps being easily induced. The excitement is often followed by a paretic [paralytic] or comatose state of depression.

The cause of this condition is still obscure, but it is probably not a simple magnesium deficiency, since pasture grass is a good source of this mineral. Young, fast-growing pasture grass on well-fertilized pastures is suspected by some to contain an unbalanced content of minerals or toxic products which cause the disease. Sjollema (*49*) believes that heavy grain feeding in winter, together with limited roughage consumption, predisposes cattle to this disease, since such rations are usually low in calcium and high in phosphorus. A condition called grass tetany is reported by Quin (*45*) to occur in Kansas, Nebraska and Oklahoma among cattle turned out to young lush pastures of rye, wheat or barley; no blood studies are reported. Metzger (*28*) states that, with few exceptions, the cases reported in Kentucky occur in cows grazing on young, rapidly growing grass and the record rainfall during the spring of 1935 caused a marked increase in the number of cases.

Since the disease is often rapidly fatal, there may not be sufficient time for treatment. Intravenous injection of a solution containing calcium chloride and magnesium chloride, which of course requires the services of a qualified veterinarian, has given good results (*49*). After the injection, it is advisable to keep the animal quiet and feed it only dry hay. Taking cattle off pasture at night for the first 2 weeks or so and giving them a feeding of hay has been recommended as a preventive measure.

Salt (Sodium Chloride) Deficiency

Such common feeds as forages, grains and grain by products ordinarily do not contain enough sodium and chlorine to meet the needs of farm animals. Milk production, hot weather and hard work with excessive sweating increase the salt requirement. Symptoms of salt deficiency in dairy cows are loss of appetite, salt hunger, rough hair coat and a rapid decline in condition and milk yield. Special attention should be given to providing an adequate supplement of salt, which may be supplied in granulated, flake, rock or block form. Animals will usually consume more in the granulated or flake than in the solid form. Potassium or sodium iodide when needed, bonemeal and ground limestone are frequently mixed together with salt and fed free choice or included in the gram mixture. On the range, boxes containing salt or general mineral mixtures should be protected from rain as much as possible and enough boxes should be supplied so that even the very timid animals will have ample opportunity to obtain some. Animals that have been deprived of salt for a considerable period should not be given all they will eat at once, but should first be hand-fed limited amounts for several days or harmful results may follow.

Potassium Deficiency in Calves

Salts of potassium are also required by the body for normal nutrition, but any practical diet usually contains an ample quantity of this mineral. Experimental semipurified rations containing 0.10 to 0.12 percent of potassium have been fed to calves, beginning at 160 days of age, by Sykes and Alfredson (*50*). They report finding lowered serum potassium, which promptly increased when additional potassium was fed, while the calcium, phosphorus and magnesium values were not altered from normal. A striking result of their studies was the finding that three of the four calves used developed marked changes in the heart, determined by the electrocardiograph. Histological (cell) changes. were also found in the Purkinje system (conducting tissue) of the right and left ventricles.

The Trace Minerals in Cattle Nutrition

Iodine Deficiency and Goiter

Iodine deficiency in cattle nutrition, as in that of other animals, is largely a sectional problem. The areas of the greatest iodine deficiency are in the Northwest and in the North Central States around the Great Lakes.

Nutritional Anemia (Iron, Copper and Cobalt Deficiency)

For many years a condition occurring in cattle in Florida, known as salt sick and a similar or identical malady in Michigan, called Grand Traverse or lake-shore disease, have caused considerable loss to the cattle industry in certain areas of these States. Affected animals gradually lose their appetites and become emaciated and weak. Some have a depraved appetite. Diarrhoea or severe constipation may be present. The blood is pale, owing to its low content of hemoglobin (red blood pigment). Young cattle fail to grow normally and if they survive do not reach normal adult size. Sexual maturity is delayed and reproduction and lactation are very unsatisfactory. After death the liver, kidneys and other tissues are pale and the heart muscle is flabby. The disease is most prevalent in young cattle over 6 months of age and in heifers calving for the first time. Cattle of all ages and both sexes may be affected when the animals are restricted to deficient ranges.

Recent studies indicate that salt-sick animals are frequently suffering from a deficiency of one or more minerals and possibly other factors also. Copper deficiency and cobalt deficiency may occur separately or overlap in some areas. In Michigan the condition is due essentially to cobalt deficiency.

Neal and Ahmann (*33*), of Florida, describe the symptoms of cobalt deficiency in calves (Fig. 3) fed a ration of natal grass hay, shelled corn and dried skim milk as follows: Affected cattle usually show a long rough coat of hair, scaliness of the skin, listlessness, retarded development of sexual characteristics, gauntness due to loss of appetite (much less marked when liquid skin milk is a part of the ration) and muscular atrophy. The erythrocyte (red blood corpuscle) count may be above average and the hemoglobin concentration equal to or above that in animals receiving cobalt and making normal growth. The amount of hemoglobin per erythrocyte or per volume of erythrocytes, is reduced. The condition would be classified as a microcytic hypochromic anemia (an anemia characterized by undersized red blood corpuscles and too little hemoglobin). The spleen is shriveled and fibrous and the heart of normal size but very flabby.

Copper deficiency also causes nutritional anemia, loss of appetite, slow growth, lowered fertility and occasionally bleaching of the hair coat in cattle. Further studies will undoubtedly yield additional information on how deficiencies of copper and cobalt and possibly of other trace minerals, may be differentiated.

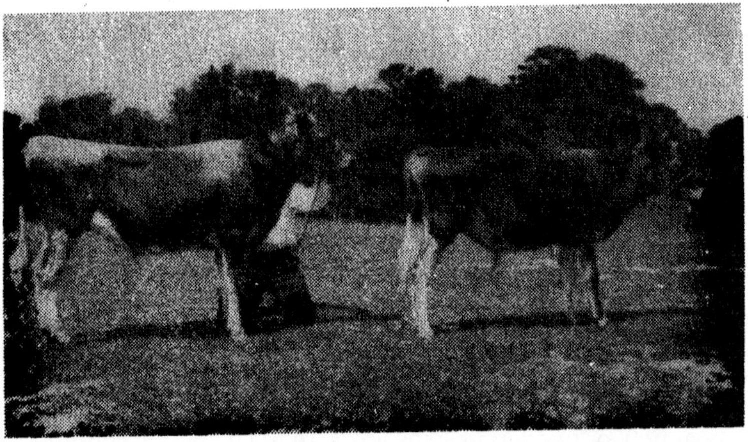

Fig. 3: These two purebred Jersey bulls were fed a ration of natal grass hay and shelled corn from cobalt-deficient land, with skim milk. The addition of 5 milligrams of cobalt daily to the ration of the animal on the left resulted in its weighing 550 pounds at 15 months of age, while the maximum weight of the animal on the right at 16 months of age was 350 pounds. (Courtesy of W.M. Neal, Florida Agricultural Experiment Station).

Workers at the Florida experiment station have demonstrated that the forage and soil are usually lower in iron, calcium, magnesium and phosphorus in areas where salt sick occurs than in areas where cattle are not affected with nutritional anemia (35). Iron deficiency has been thought to be a cause of this disease, but recent studies tend to give more weight to the possibility of a deficiency of cobalt or copper or both.[4] In Michigan the cobalt content of the hay grown in affected areas is considerably lower than that of hay from forms where the disease does not develop.

---

[4] Communication to the Animal Nutrition Division from W.M. Neal, of the Florida Agricultural Experiment Station.

Considerable success has been attained in treating and preventing anemia in cattle by supplying iron, cobalt or copper salts along with common salt for use as a lick. Advanced cases have also been successfully treated by drenching animals with these salts in solution. There is some indication that the responses obtained from feeding iron salts are due at least in part to the cobalt impurity which these salts frequently contain. Cases of Grand Traverse disease in Michigan respond well to a cobalt supplement alone (3).

In Florida supplements of 5 to 10 milligrams of cobalt a day markedly improved the growth of calves on a cobalt-deficient ration. Calves fed supplements of ferric ammonium sulfate and copper sulfate developed deficiency symptoms sooner than individuals on the basal ration only, while those receiving supplements of cobalt or of iron, copper and cobalt appeared normal (*34*). Cobalt deficiency in the feeds of Florida is associated with certain soil types (Norfolk series) low in cobalt; it may also be associated with copper deficiency.

Whenever salt-sick cattle fail to respond to the usual supplement of iron and copper, it has been recommended by the Florida Agricultural Experiment Station[5] that cobalt be added to the mineral mixture.

For advanced cases the following treatment is recommended:

Dissolve 10 grams of cobalt chloride or cobalt sulfate in one gallon of water. Give mature animals 6 ounces * * * as a drench once weekly for three or four weeks. Calves should be given 3 ounces and other animals in proportion.

For prevention of the disease:

Add one pound of cobalt chloride or cobalt sulfate to each ton of the regular salt sick mixture (100 lbs. of salt, 25 lbs. of red oxide of iron and 1 lb. of powdered copper sulfate). A recommended manner of making this addition is to dissolve 22 grams of the cobalt salt in a small amount of water and spray it over 100 lbs. of the salt sick mineral with a fly sprayer or atomizer. It should be mixed thoroughly so that animals taking it will secure a uniform amount. This should be offered in protected mineral boxes at all times.

---

[5] COBALT IN THE TREATMENT AND PREVENTION OF SALT SICK. Fla. Agr. Expt. Sta. [1] p; 1937. [Processed].

Toxic Minerals

Selenium and Fluorine Poisoning

Losses due to consumption of plants containing toxic amounts of selenium occur among livestock on the ranges and ranch lands of the Great Plains, particularly in South Dakota, Wyoming and Nebraska. Other States that undoubtedly have a more or less serious selenium problem are North Dakota, Kansas, Oklahoma, Texas, New Mexico, Arizona, Colorado, Utah and Montana.

Symptoms of chronic poisoning are described by Moxon (*32*).

An acute attack may lead to so-called blind staggers, as commonly reported from Wyoming. This name for the disease is misleading, since the animals do not always become blind or stagger, but they do have a tendency to stray, stumble over objects in their way and bump into objects and attempt to push them over rather than walk around them. In the last stages paralysis may set in and the animal dies with symptoms of abdominal pain, grinding of the teeth and respiratory failure.

Prevention of selenium poisoning involves keeping animals away from areas that produce toxic plants, not always an easy matter.

Treatment of alkali disease or blind staggers, is not entirely successful, since the injury caused by selenium is often permanent. The Wyoming station (*4*) reports success in treating blind staggers in the early stages by hypodermic injections of strychnine and drenching with warm water. The treatment should be carried out by a competent veterinarian. Changing the ration of the animal to selenium-free grain, a protein-rich concentrate and good hay will do much to favor recovery if the damage to the internal organs has not been too great. Recent work at the South Dakota experiment station indicates that small amounts of arsenic (12 to 15 parts per million) in the feed or drinking water are effective in treating selenium poisoning in cattle as well as in dogs and chickens.

Fluorine poisoning in cattle is most frequently the result of feeding such products as raw phosphatic limestone as a mineral supplement. A purified product low in fluorine is now available for livestock feeding.

Fluorine poisoning as seen in cattle is usually of the chronic type caused by the consumption of a small amount of fluorine over a considerable period. In mineral-feeding investigations with dairy cattle, Reed and Huffman (*46*), of Michigan and Phillips, Hart and Bohstedt (*42*), of Wisconsin, have observed the harmful effects of feeding raw rock phosphate in amounts ranging from 0.625 percent to 2.5 percent of the grain mixture. In the Michigan studies the health of the animals declined and their teeth became badly worn. The condition of the teeth was first discovered when the animals were about 2½ years of age. At this time the animals began to lap cold water when drinking; if the water was warmed to body temperature they would drink freely. The jawbones and leg bones became abnormally thick and rough. Other symptoms noted were loss of appetite, progressive emaciation, decreased milk yield, delay of estrum after parturition and lowered birth weight of calves. These may have been secondary effects due to the poor condition of the animals.

Animals usually recover to some extent if the period of fluorine feeding has not been too long and damage to the body is not too severe. The source of excessive fluorine in the ration should be removed. Cattle with excessively worn and defective teeth have difficulty in eating dried roughage but many improve considerably if turned out to pasture.

Vitamin-Deficiency Diseases of Cattle

Cattle and other ruminants are unique among animals in their vitamin requirements. According to present knowledge., vitamin A or its precursor, carotene and vitamin D are the only vitamins that must be furnished in order to prevent characteristic nutritional diseases. Nearly all of the recognized vitamin B factors are known to be synthesized by bacteria in the digestive tract of these animals, but information is still lacking on whether this source is entirely adequate under an conditions. Vitamin C is also synthesized in the body by cattle. Recent studies have indicated that under certain conditions the formation of vitamin C may be inadequate, but under such circumstances a dietary source of vitamin C is apparently of no benefit and injection of the vitamin appears necessary to maintain successful reproduction. Most cattle feeds are rich in vitamin E, but there is no conclusive evidence that this vitamin is essential.

Fortunately most cattle feeds such as green pasture grass, hay, silage of good quality and cereal grains are rich in the known vitamins. The essential vitamins should be furnished to cattle in ordinary feeds whenever possible. An understanding of the conditions under which vitamin deficiencies are likely to occur and prompt recognition of early symptoms of deficiency are essential to eliminate, the large losses caused by these diseases.

Vitamin A Deficiency

Vitamin A deficiency is the most common vitamin-deficiency disease of cattle (*18*). It has been reported from the Southern States, where cottonseed meal and hulls are fed, from the West and Southwest, where large numbers of cattle are grazed on ranges that become deficient in carotene-rich forage because of drought or overstocking and from the Midwest and sections where corn or cereal grains, beet by products, cereal hay and straw or old hay or poorly cured forage are used to fatten cattle. The practice of wintering cattle in stubble-fields with access to a straw stack without a supplement of well-cured hay which has retained a good green color may also lead to a deficiency of this vitamin, particularly in young, growing cattle or pregnant animals.

Symptoms of vitamin A deficiency appear in cattle of all ages after they have been for an extended period on a ration containing too little carotene or vitamin A. One of the first symptoms of the deficiency that can be detected in fattening cattle or adult animals is night blindness or an inability of the animals to see well in dim light, as during the late evening. This can be detected by driving the cattle about in a corral and noting whether they bump into the fence or each other or stumble over objects placed in their way. Several stages or degrees of night blindness can be recognized and the condition may progress to total blindness unless the deficiency is corrected.

Night blindness results from inability of the animal to regenerate sufficient visual purple, a light-sensitive pigment of the retina, which is a compound of vitamin A and a protein. In young animals night blindness may progress rapidly to permanent blindness owing to injury to the optic nerve. Simple night blindness can usually be cured, but injury to the optic nerve is likely to result in permanent damage. In the advanced stages of vitamin A deficiency the eye is very sensitive to bright light. Animals are somewhat dazzled, blinking abnormally or keeping their eyes closed when exposed to bright sunlight. An excessive secretion of tears, which run out over the face and jaw, is often seen. In total blindness the pupil is fully dilated and in some cases the cornea may ulcerate or become opaque.

Swelling of the legs and forequarters (commonly called anasarca) is often found in cattle showing symptoms of vitamin A deficiency (Fig. 4). This condition has been observed in a large number of fat cattle coming from the Corn Belt in the Middle West. Other symptoms noted in this condition are rapid respiration, stiffness or lameness, night blindness, total blindness, convulsions, loss of appetite and loss of weight. Death occurs in advanced cases. When such animals are slaughtered, an extensive edema (warlogged condition) of the fat and muscle tissues is found, a condition that occurs in dry-lot-fed cattle that have been on low-carotene rations for 10 to 18 months or longer. The animals recover within a few weeks if well-cured alfalfa hay is added to the ration (*11*).

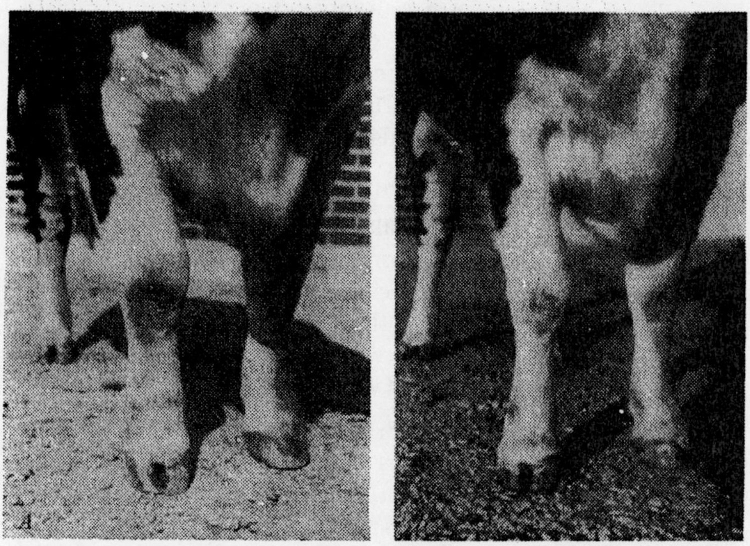

Fig. 4: ***A*: Swelling (generalized edema, or anasarca) of the legs, brisket, and shoulders is often associated with vitamin A deficiency; *B*: after liberal doses of vitamin A or a ration of well-cured hay the edema usually disappears.**

Cows and bulls may lose their reproductive ability in advanced vitamin A deficiency, but the interruption of sexual activity or damage to the sexual organs is not always permanent. The usual course is for the cows to conceive and later to either abort or give birth to weak or blind calves, which often fail to survive. Cows that have deficient calves may remain apparently normal themselves, even though they are receiving an insufficient amount of carotene for normal reproduction. Hart and Guilbert (*19*) report that retention of the placenta is common in vitamin-A-deficient cows.

Calves suffer from vitamin A deficiency within a few weeks after birth unless their ration is adequate in this factor. Calves deficient at birth are often blind and weak, slow to get up and very wobbly on their legs. They may have convulsions shortly after birth and these often continue intermittently with increasing severity until death (Fig. 5). Such calves frequently suffer from diarrhoea (or occasionally constipation) and may develop respiratory disorders such as pneumonia. Blindness usually develops in the later stages. As the deficiency progresses, the coat becomes rough, the appetite is poor and growth is slow or there is loss in weight. Examination of calves that die from vitamin A deficiency usually reveals that blindness is due to stenosis of the optic nerve (*29*), while a cystic pituitary with considerable destruction of glandular tissue 6 and white spotted kidneys (*30*) may also be found.

Cause, Prevention and Treatment

All inadequate carotene intake over a period long enough to permit almost complete exhaustion of the body stores of preformed vitamin A and carotene is the principal cause of vitamin A deficiency in cattle. Since for age, either fresh or cured, is the chief source of carotene for cattle, the kind, quality and amount of forage consumed are the first factors to investigate if vitamin A deficiency is suspected.

During extended periods of drought, pasture and range herbage becomes scarce and is also lower than usual in carotene, protein and phosphorus. Consequently cattle grazing under such conditions are subjected to a short- age of carotene and other essential factors. Carotene deficiency is an important economic problem in the West, South and Southwest where large numbers of beef cattle

---

[6] MADSEN, LOUIS L., HALL, S.R., AND CONVERSE, H.T. Unpublished data, Bur. Anim. Indus. and Bur. Dairy Indus.

are grazed on ranges which may become deficient in carotene containing forage because of insufficient rainfall. Feeder cattle raised under these conditions may show symptoms of vitamin A, deficiency or have such a low body storage of vitamin A and carotene that they develop this deficiency later during I the fattening period.

In work of the Bureau of Animal Industry in cooperation with the Texas Agricultural Experiment Station it was found that the time required for the development of night blindness in cattle fed a carotene - deficient ration varied considerably, depending on the age of the animals and their previous nutritional history. Older animals on carotene-rich feeds accumulate a larger supply of carotene than younger animals and consequently deficiency symptoms appear first in the young animals on a vitamin-A-deficient diet. During grazing seasons of abundant rainfall all animals have a larger storage of carotene than during periods of drought. In this work, reported by Riggs (47), yearling steer calves showed symptoms of vitamin A depletion within 128 to 266 days, with an average of 178 ± 37 days, while younger calves (3 to 5 months old) developed night blindness within 46 to 61 days during 1939 and steers of the same age developed these symptoms within 65 to 131 days during 1939-40. In work of the Bureau of Animal Industry at Beltsville, Md., symptoms of vitamin A deficiency became evident in a group of yearling Hereford heifers as early as 60 days after they came off good pasture and were given a carotene-deficient ration.

Carotene requirements for fattening beef cattle have been investigated at the Texas Agricultural Experiment Station in cooperation with the Bureau of Animal Industry. Steer calves used in the experiments were first largely depleted of their vitamin A reserves and were then divided into five groups and fed sufficient alfalfa-leaf meal at five levels of carotene intake so as to provide 1,250 to 5,000 micrograms of carotene per 100 pounds of body weight daily. No significant differences were found in rate of gain, carcass weight or carcass grade after a 140-day fattening period. Steers fed the 1,250- and 1,500-microgram level remained completely night blind and night blindness persisted in some of the steers fed the 2,500- and 3,000-microgram levels. Steers fed 5,000 micrograms of carotene per 100 pounds of body weight became essentially normal.

The condition of fattening animals is not necessarily an indication of inadequate carotene intake, since animals may be

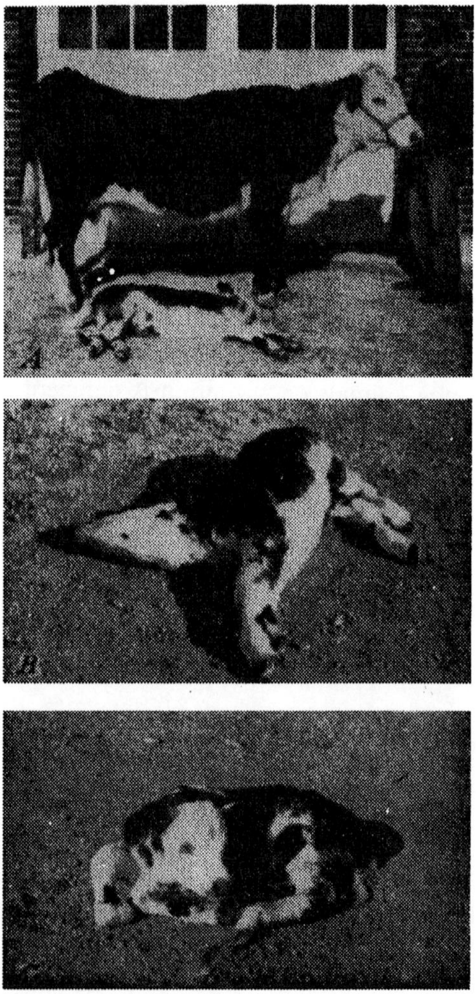

Fig. 5: If a cow's ration is low in carotene during the gestation period, her calf may be blind and weak at birth. *A*: This cow is in good condition and shows no evidence of vitamin A deficiency other than low blood carotene and vitamin A. Her calf was normal in size and condition but was unable to stand alone and had frequent convulsions. *B*: shows the characteristic attitude during a convulsions. *C*: Abnormal position of front legs. This calf could not stand alone until 4 days of age and survived only 4 weeks.

critically low in this factor and yet appear to be in good condition. This deficiency never occurs in cattle fattened on good pasture, but it should be guarded against in lot-fed cattle receiving heavy rations of grain with roughages of relatively low carotene content. Vitamin A deficiency can be avoided or corrected in fattening cattle by feeding at least 2 to 3 pounds of new green, leafy (preferably legume) hay daily to each animal.

Carotene or vitamin A requirements for normal reproduction are much higher than for the prevention of night blindness or other common symptoms of vitamin A deficiency. For dairy cattle, Converse and Meigs[7] found that normal calvings resulted when timothy, clover or alfalfa hay was fed without pasture if the hay was of high quality and rich in carotene. In a limited number of experiments a carotene intake of 80 to 100 milligrams appeared sufficient and a daily intake of 50 to 60 milligrams resulted in the birth of many weak or dead calves. They point out that in order for clover and timothy hay to be graded U.S. No. 1 the hay must have 45 percent or more of green color. Carotene analyses made during these studies at Beltsville on clover and timothy hay with 50 percent of green color (slightly more than is required for U.S. No. 1) resulted in values of 18 to 20 milligrams of carotene per kilogram (2.2 pounds) of hay. Under the conditions of the experiment, it is estimated that 4½ kilograms (about 10 pounds) of this high-quality hay daily would supply sufficient carotene for normal reproduction.

In some preliminary studies by Davis and Madsen (*12a*), 60 micro- grams of carotene per kilogram of body weight (about 2,727 micrograms per 100 pounds of body weight) was found to be sufficient for beef heifers to produce calves which were apparently normal at birth. Calves born to beef heifers receiving 30 and 45 micrograms of carotene per kilogram of body weight were weak or blind at birth and had other symptoms of vitamin A deficiency.

Work in the Bureau of Dairy Industry at Beltsville, Md., has also shown that the minimum amount of carotene and vitamin A needed for the cure of night blindness in cattle does not furnish enough for

---

[7] CONVERSE, H.T., and MEIGS, EDWARD B. THE CAROTENE REQUIREMENTS OF DAIRY CATTLE FOR NORMAL REPRODUCTION. U.S. Bur. Dairy Indus. BDIM-827, [4] pp. 1938: [Processed].

normal growth and health in young calves. The vitamin A needs of calves are summarized by Converse and Meigs,[8] as follows:

The experiment shows:

(1) That when skim milk is fed even after a month on whole milk, calves should receive some well-cured green hay as a source of vitamin A unless cod-liver oil or some other supplement is furnished;

(2) That too much dependence should not be placed on whole milk feeding to supply vitamin A unless the milk comes from cows on pasture;

(3) That milk does vary widely enough in its vitamin A content to indicate needed caution in its selection for calf feeding;

(4) That whole milk in the calf ration is needed more for its vitamin A content than for its fat or energy; and

(5) That 20 to 25 cubic centimeters of animal-feeding cod-liver oil or 15 milligrams of carotene roughly equals the vitamin A requirement of growing calves during the milk-feeding age.

Feeds low in carotene, which should be supplemented with carotene-rich feeds if fed to cattle over an extended period, are cottonseed meal and hulls, linseed and soybean meals, wheat, oats, barley, corn (white or yellow), sorghum grains, beet pulp and molasses, cereal straw, corn stover, low-grade legume or grass hays, range herbage during extended periods of drought and hays held in storage more than 1 year. Feeds rich in carotene are green pasture (grass, legume or browse), high-grade green, leafy hay (legume, grass or cereal) of the current year's crop, well-made silage (corn, grass or legume) and new high-grade alfalfa meal.

The Vitamin B Complex in Bovine Nutrition

Interest concerning the role of the vitamin B complex in the nutrition of cattle dates back to the early work of Theiler and associates in South Africa (52), reported in 1915. They suggested

---

[8] CONVERSE, H.T., and MEIGS, EDWARD B. CAROTENE AND VITAMIN A IN THE NUTRITION OF DAIRY CALVES. U.S. Bur. Dairy Indus. BDIM-645, 4 pp. 1934. [Processed].

after some rice-feeding experiments in which small amounts of roughage were also fed that:

> It may be that cattle are capable of synthesizing their own vitamins in virtue of the extensive bacterial flora of their intestinal tract–a sort of commensal symbiosis.

This hypothesis was investigated later by workers at the Pennsylvania experiment station (*5*) and was shown to be true for what was then called vitamin B. The workers were successful in obtaining apparently normal growth, gestation and parturition in dairy heifers on a ration that was low in vitamin B as determined by rat growth. Successful lactation was never obtained for more than several weeks, however. The reason for failure in lactation has never been satisfactorily explained. The work was carried out before the complex nature or chemical properties of the vitamin B group were known. Recent work has confirmed the original observation of vitamin synthesis in the digestive tract of ruminants and considerable information is now available on the formation of the individual members of the B complex.

The question whether synthesis of the vitamin B complex in the digestive tract of cattle is sufficient to meet their needs under all circumstances has not been solved in all details. The report from the Kenya Colony (*12*) that "sweating sickness" in calves, characterized by clinical symptoms similar to those of blacktongue in dogs and pellagra in human beings, is interesting in this regard. Rapid recovery from this disease follows treatment with bakers' yeast or liver extract. Newman and Savage (*36*) have noted improved results by including dried brewers' yeast and cereal-yeast feed in a dry calf starter fed to young calves that received a limited amount of milk. Baker (*2*) describes beneficial results from feeding yeast to calves that were in an advanced state of malnutrition and debility as a result of diarrhoea; followed by constipation and loss of appetite due to gastrointestinal parasitism (trichostrongylosis). After the animals had gained in appetite and strength, anthelmintic (worm) treatment was successfully administered and the animals made remarkable recoveries.

Fortunately most feeds of good quality commonly used in cattle feeding are usually good sources of most of the individual vitamins of the B complex. Circumstances may upset their intake however and other conditions such as infectious diseases, heavy gastrointestinal parasitism or other disturbances may have a modifying influence on the synthesis of essential factors in the digestive tract. More research on this subject is necessary.

Vitamin C (Ascorbic Acid) and Breeding Efficiency

It has been the belief for a long time that farm animals as a group, including poultry, usually synthesize enough vitamin C to meet their requirements, but recent studies indicate that this is not always true. Phillips and coworkers (*44*), at the Wisconsin station, have shown that calves on a carotene-deficient ration do not maintain normal levels of vitamin C in their blood plasma or urine. Later work (*43*) indicated that the breeding efficiency of some bulls with low fertility could be markedly improved by subcutaneous injections of ascorbic acid. Directions for ascorbic acid therapy of slow-breeding bulls have recently been published (*41*). The average dose recommended is 5 milligrams of ascorbic acid per kilogram (2.2 pounds) of body weight or 1 to 2 grams per 1,000 pounds of body weight injected at 3- to 4-day intervals for 5 or 6 weeks or until the bull shows improvement. Preliminary work also indicates that vitamin C treatment of cows that fail to conceive may also be beneficial in some cases (*1*).

Vitamin D Deficiency

Vitamin D is essential for normal calcium and phosphorus metabolism in both young and adult cattle. Vitamin D deficiency is most apt to occur during the winter season, when the sun's rays are less potent in ultraviolet light or during periods of barn feeding when the animals do not have access to either sunshine or sun-cured roughage. Bone deformities are probably the most easily recognized feature of the nutritional disease; however, vitamin D deficiency leads to important changes in the body fluids and other tissues also. Vitamin D deficiency in cattles very rare except under experimental conditions.

Vitamin D in any form is suitable for the cure or prevention of rickets in calves. Duncan and Huffman (*13, 21*) have demonstrated the effectiveness of sunshine and sun-cured roughage in curing and preventing rickets experimentally produced in calves. One to two pounds of sun-cured alfalfa a day prevented rickets in calves up to 195 days of age. However, in work at the Pennsylvania experiment station (*7*) 1 pound of sun-cured alfalfa did not have sufficient antirachitic potency to produce a well-calcified skeleton in young calves kept away from direct sunshine over a 6-month feeding period. Two pounds of good sun-cured timothy a day was found to prevent rickets up to 1 year of age, while 3 pounds of hay cured rickets in an animal at 9 months of age. Bechtel and associates (*8*) found that calves would not eat enough corn silage to prevent rickets when an experimental basal ration low in vitamin D was fed, but that in older animals consuming 15 to 20 pounds of silage rachitic symptoms were alleviated in 3 out of 4 cases. Bechdel and coworkers (*6, 7*) found that 3 to 5 pounds of oat straw or 2½ pounds of sun-cured alfalfa prevented rickets, while up to 2½ pounds of night-harvested, machine-dried alfalfa or alfalfa machine-dried immediately after cutting in the day-time was ineffective. Ultraviolet irradiation of the basal ration or irradiation of the calves themselves cured rickets, while feeding cod-liver-oil concentrate or irradiated yeast at the rate of 300 U.S.P. units of vitamin D per 100 pounds of body weight or more per day prevented rickets in calves from birth to 7 months of age. Long, Huffman and Duncan (*23*) found that only 0.3 to 0.4 U.S.P. units of vitamin D per pound of body weight was necessary to prevent rickets in the growing calf when winter and early spring milk was the sole source of vitamin D, if normal plasma magnesium values were maintained.

Daily exposure to the sun during the summer protects calves against rickets, but during cloudy weather in the late fall and winter extra vitamin D may be needed if roughage of low quality is fed and if the calves are kept inside for long periods because of bad weather. The vitamin D requirements of adult cattle can be readily satisfied by regular exposure to sunshine, together with a liberal amount of sun-cured roughage as normally fed in practical rations.

Vitamin E and Sterility in Cattle

Benefits from wheat-germ oil (rich in vitamin E) in the treatment of non-infectious barrenness of cattle has been reported particularly under certain feeding conditions found in Denmark and elsewhere but supporting data are rather meager and often conflicting. Under conditions in the United States, wheat-germ-oil treatment for sterility in cows has produced some confusing results. The Oregon experiment station reports (*10*):

Extensive experiments have been made to test the value of giving cows injections of the antisterility vitamin E which is being extensively advertised as somewhat of a cure-all for difficult breeding. Although earlier trials have indicated these might have some value, further and more extensive tests, using herds at the state hospitals in Salem and Pendleton, have given results too indefinite for conclusions to be drawn.

Research workers have not been able to establish satisfactorily that vitamin E is a dietary essential of calves, cows or bulls. The technical difficulties and expense involved in preparing vitamin-E-free experimental diets in the quantities needed have limited the studies with cattle.

Since most cattle feeds are good sources of vitamin E, a natural deficiency of the vitamin in balanced rations would, of course, normally be rare (*20, 40*).

Determination of the need of including vitamin-E-rich concentrates in cattle rations in order to insure fertility and overcome certain forms of sterility awaits further work.

Miscellaneous Nutritional Diseases and Disorders of Cattle

Urinary Calculi (Urolithiasis)

Cattle frequently suffer from the formation of crystalline deposits or stonelike concretions in the urinary tract. The size, number and location of the calculi mainly determine whether or not symptoms of the condition become evident.

Newsom (*37*) summarizes some of the causes of urinary calculi and discusses them under the headings of water, vitamin A, mineral unbalance, reaction, hyperparathyroidism (over activity of the parathyroid gland), infection and urinary irritation. It is evident from the list of factors that may influence calculi formation that the problem is complex. Evidence that dietary factors are concerned is definite, but it should be kept in mind that other factors may be involved and also that there are many different types and kinds of calculi.

Newsom points but that calculi are more common in winter, when water is limited or lacking because of freezing weather. The case for vitamin A deficiency as a cause of calculi formation in cattle is not complete, although some rations that tend to favor calculi formation may be low in this factor. An unbalanced mineral intake, particularly of calcium, phosphorus and magnesium, is believed to influence calculi formation in cattle to a considerable degree.

In cooperative experiments of the Bureau of Animal Industry and the Texas Agricultural Experiment Station conducted at Big Spring, Tex., a serious calculi problem has developed in steers fattened on milo grain, cottonseed meal and sorgo silage. Such rations are naturally high in magnesium. Steers given high levels of calcium, furnished either as pulverized oyster shell or bonemeal had fewer calculi than those receiving less calcium and more magnesium. The work is being continued, with special emphasis on the ratio and quantity of calcium, phosphorus and magnesium in the diet.

Bloat

Bloat is a troublesome disorder of cattle that is often the cause of heavy losses. The disease is usually of a sporadic nature; when due to overeating or consuming spoiled feeds, it may be considered as nutritional; but other conditions, such as occlusion of the openings of the forestomachs with hair balls or other foreign bodies and factors that interfere with normal rumination and intestinal movements, may also be involved. Bloating may occur suddenly or may appear in some individuals more or less regularly after each feeding.

Bloat is due to an excessive accumulation in the rumen of gases probably formed to a large extent by bacterial action. The conditions that favor the kind and amount of gas produced in the rumen and the factors that inhibit its normal removal are not completely, understood. Recent studies have indicated that the pressure of the gas in the rumen, which results in a distention of the organ, causing pressure on other vital organs such as the heart and lungs, is not the sole cause of death in bloated animals. Adsorption of toxic gases from the rumen also produces distressing symptoms and may cause death (*38*).

A number of precautions for controlling or preventing bloat have been advocated, but practically none have proved to be of much value under experimental tests. It is generally agreed, however, that legume pastures (alfalfa, clovers, etc.) are more likely to cause bloating than is grass. A young, lush growth of legumes appears to be more dangerous than the mature forage. Pasture that is wet with dew is often said to be particularly dangerous. Before turning hungry animals on legume pasture, it may be worth while to give them a good feed of dry hay so they will not gorge themselves on green forage.

It is possible that soil conditions under which a feed is grown may also influence its tendency to produce bloat. McIntosh (*24*) states that:

The farmers who have the least trouble with bloating are those whose alfalfa fields are in a high state of fertility, while those who have the greatest amount of trouble are farmers whose pasture land is in a worn-out condition.

His theory has not been critically tested, but it is no doubt worthy of careful consideration. The determination of the chemical characteristics of feeds that cause bloat and a more accurate definition of the environmental and physiological factors concerned in this disease are important problems for further study.

Fattening cattle or heavy-milking cows that receive large quantities of grain also have a tendency to bloat. In cattle-fattening experiments, Osland and coworkers (*39*) at the Colorado experiment station report that:

* * * barley, when fed alone in a grain, cottonseed cake and hay ration, is not a safe feed for calves because of its tendency to cause bloat, even though it is fed at the rate of only 1 percent of their live weight or less. The addition of cheap, bulky carbonaceous feeds such as wet beet pulp, silage or potatoes has proved effective in checking digestive troubles but has failed to prevent bloats entirely.

Similar results were obtained by the Bureau of Animal Industry in cooperation with the Montana experiment station. A large proportion of steer calves fattened on barley and alfalfa were found to suffer from bloat or other digestive disturbances that caused scouring or going off feed. Feeding a gram ration consisting of an equal amount of barley and dried molasses-beet pulp, however, resulted in no serious cases of bloat or other digestive disorders. In these experiments bloat was usually treated by drenching the animals with as much as 12 ounces of raw linseed oil.

In severe cases of bloat, puncturing the paunch with a trocar may be necessary. This operation may injure the animal if not done properly and it should be performed by a qualified veterinarian whenever possible. Further treatment to stop fermentation in the paunch and restore normal gastrointestinal activity may also be prescribed.

Ketosis

The metabolic disorder of cattle in which there is an abnormal quantity of ketone bodies (acetone, acetoacetic acid and betahydroxybutyric acid) in the blood, urine and milk is an important problem in the dairy industry. The disease causes a loss of condition in affected animals, a marked decline in milk flow and the production of a characteristic off-flavored milk. Duncan, Huffman and Tobin (*15*) studied this condition in a herd of Jersey cows under farm conditions, many of which were seriously affected with the disease. The disorder was apparently associated with feeding a ration of poor-quality soybean hay, corn silage and a small amount of grain during the fall and winter. The disease was described as follows:

> The occurrence of the disturbance in the health and milk production of the cows became most pronounced within two to six weeks following a normal parturition. It was the owner's opinion that the cows were in good nutritional condition before calving and that all had begun to produce large quantities of milk. He also observed that the cows lost appetite gradually, rapidly decreased in milk production, became constipated, hide-bound, listless and emaciated in appearance. He reported that the barn had a peculiar odor at times.
>
> Cows in the most critical condition were given chloral hydrate (1 dram in 12 ounces of warm water 3 times a day for 1 day) and this was repeated later in severe cases. The ration of all the animals was changed. Liberal quantities of alfalfa hay of medium quality and cornstalks were fed instead of the soybean hay and silage previously used. Severely affected cows were given 1 to 2 pounds of corn sugar or molasses and the grain was increased to 5 pounds a day. The new feeding schedule resulted in marked improvement within 2 weeks in most cases, as shown by improvement in appetite and general condition and by a decrease of the ketone bodies in the blood, urine and milk as determined by chemical analyses.

Duncan and coworkers and others have reached the general conclusion that ketosis may be reduced in small-fed animals by feeding hay of a good quality together with a liberal supply of grain. In addition, high producing individuals should have some feed that is a source of quickly available sugar, such as molasses. Turning animals to pasture also resulted in recovery. An extract from the anterior lobe of the pituitary and even vitamin B_1, have been reported to be of use in the treatment of this disease.

Overeating and Undernutrition

Cattle, like other farm animals, are adversely affected by overeating. When this occurs, the regular ration, except water, should 1 be withheld for a day or two and they should be slowly brought back on feed, a small amount of palatable roghage being given first, with gradual introduction of the grain mixture as the appetite returns. If there is severe constipation after an attack of diarrhoea, it should be treated as soon as possible with Epsom salts, raw linseed oil or pure mineral oil. The advice and help of a qualified veterinarian may prevent serious consequences if it is obtained early enough.

Lactating dairy cows are occasionally overfed when record-breaking production is desired. Symptoms of overeating are loss of appetite, dullness, diarrhoea, distention of the rumen (bloat) and a marked drop in the milk yield. Milk fever occurs most often In heavily fed, high-producing animals. In an effort to force apparently normal animals to maximum performance or above, drugs are occasionally prescribed to stimulate appetite, a practice that should be discouraged. The record may be attained, but the productive life and reproductive ability of the animal may thereby be permanently injured. Losses due to overeating can best be controlled or prevented by careful feeding, with strict attention to the appetites of the animals.

Underfeeding may be harmful to the animal body and is frequently uneconomical (27). Under nutrition may come from either quantitative or qualitative deficiencies in the ration or from both.

Losses from livestock consuming poisonous plants on the range are usually largest during periods of drought or when the range is overgrazed. Shortage of water is as serious or more so than a lack of feed. Forsling (*16*) discusses the dangers of overstocking.

Hart (*17*) points out that "profitable livestock management does not include allowing animals to border on starvation or failure to supply sufficient quantities of essential substances until symptoms appear."

Literature Cited

(1) ANONYMOUS. (1940). "HARD TO SETTLE" COWS RESPOND TO VITAMIN INJECTIONS. Wis. Agr. Expt. Sta. Ann. Rept. (Bul. 450): 37-38, in us.

(2) BAKER, DONALD W. (1941). YEAST AS AN ADJUNCT TO THE ANTHELMINTIC TREATMENT OF ADVANCED CASES OF TRICHOSTRONGYLOSIS IN CALVES. Cornell Vet. 31: 13-16.

(3) BALTZER, A.C., KILLHAM, B.J., DUNCAN, C.W. and HUFFMAN, C.F. (1941). A COBALT DEFICIENCY DISEASE OBSERVED IN SOME MICHIGAN CATTLE. Mich. Agr. Expt. Sta. Quart. Bul. 24: 68-70.

(4) BEATH, O.A., DRAIZE, J.H. and GILBERT, C.S. (1934). PLANTS POISONOUS TO LIVESTOCK. Wyo. Agr. Expt. Sta. Bul. 200, 84 pp., illus.

(5) BECHDEL, S.I., ECKLES, C.H. and PALMER, L.S. (1926). THE VITAMIN B REQUIREMENT OF THE CALF. Jour. Dairy Sci. 9: 409-438, illus.

(6) ______HILSTON, W.W., GUERRANT, N.B. and DUTCHER. R.A. (1938). THE VITAMIN D REQUIREMENT OF DAIRY CALVES. Pa. Agr. Expt. Sta. Bul. 364, 26 pp., illus.

(7) ______LANDSBURG, K.G. and HILL, O. J. (1933). RICKETS IN CALVES. Pa. Agr. Expt. Sta. Tech. Bul. 291, 41 pp., illus.

(8) BECHTEL, H. ERNEST, HUFFMAN, C.F., DUNCAN, C.W. and HOPPERT, C.A. (1936). VITAMIN D STUDIES IN CATTLE, IV. CORN SILAGE AS A SOURCE OF VITAMIN D FOR DAIRY CATTLE. Jour. Dairy Sci. 19: 359-372.

(9) BECKER, R.B., NEAL, W.M. and SHEALY, A.L. (1934). EFFECT OF CALCIUM-DEFICIENT ROUGHAGES UPON MILK YIELD AND BONE STRENGTH IN CATTLE. Jour. Dairy Sci. 17: 1-10, illus.

(10) BESSE, RALPH S. (1938)DAIRY CATTLE DISEASES. Oreg. Agr. Expt. Sta. Bien. Rpt. 1936-38 (Bul. 359): 58-59.

(11) CREECH, G.T. and MADSEN, L.L. (1942). GENERALIZED EDEMA OR THE SO-CALLED ANASARCA IN CATTLE. Bur. Vet. 18: 1-3, illus.

(12) DAUBNEY, R. (1936). REPORT OF THE CHIEF VETERINARY RESEARCH OFFICER FOR THE YEAR 1934: SWEATING SICKNESS IN CALVES. Kenya Colony Dept. Agr. Ann. Rpt. 3: 31-32.

(12a)DAVIS, RUSSELL E. and MADSEN, LOUIS I. (1941). CAROTENE AND VITAMIN A IN CATTLE BLOOD PLASMA, WITH OBSERVATIONS ON REPRODUCTIVE PERFORMANCE AT RESTRICTED LEVELS OF CAROTENE INTAKE. Jour. Nutr. 21: 135-146, illus.

(13) DUNCAN, C.W. and HUFFMAN. C.F. (1936). VITAMIN D STUDIES IN CATTLE. III. INFLUENOE OF SOLAR ULTRAVIOLET RADIATION UPON THE BLOOD CHEMISTRY AND MINERAL, METABOLISM OF DAIRY CALVES. Jour. Dairy Sci. 19: 291-303.

(14) DUNCAN, C.W., HUFFMAN, C.F. and ROBINSON, C.F. (1935). MAGNESIUM STUDIES IN CALVES. I. TETANY PRODUCED BY A RATION OF MILK OR MILK WITH VARIOUS SUPPLEMENTS. Jour. Biol. Chem. 108: 35-44.

(15) ______HUFFMAN, C.F. and TOBIN, H.A. (1939). A CHEMICAL STUDY OF KETOSIS IN A DAIRY HERD. Amer. Vet. Med. Assoc. Jour. 95: 690-700.

(16) FORSLING, C.L. (1924). SAVING LIVESTOCK FROM STARVATION ON SOUTH-WESTERN RANGES. U.S. Dept. Agr. Farmers' Bul. 1428, 22 pp., illus.

(17) HART, GEORGE H. (1938). DIETARY DEFICIENCIES AND RELATED SYMPTOMATOLOGY IN DOMESTIC ANIMALS. Amer. Vet. Med. Assoc. Jour. 92: 503-515.

(18) ______(1940). VITAMIN A DEFICIENCY AND REQUIREMENTS OF FARM MAMMALS. Nutr. Abs. and Rev. 10: [261]-272.

(19) ______and GUILBERT, H.R. (1933). VITAMIN-A DEFICIENCY AS RELATED TO REPRODUCTION IN RANGE CATTLE. Calif. Agr. Expt. Sta. Bul. 560, 30 pp., illus.

(20) HATHAWAY, I.L. and DAVIS, H.P. (1934). THE VITAMIN E CONTENT OF CERTAIN DAIRY FEEDS. Nebr. Agr. Expt. Sta. Res. Bul. 73. 7 pp.

(21) HUFFMAN, C.F. and DUNCAN, C.W. (1935). VITAMIN D STUDIES IN CATTLE. I. THE ANTIRACHITIC VALUE OF HAY IN THE RATION OF DAIRY CATTLE. Jour. Dairy Sci. 18: 511-526.

(22) ______and DUNCAN, C.W. (1936). MAGNESIUM CARBONATE AND MAGNESIUM OXIDE SUPPLEMENTS TO A WHOLE MILK RATION FOR DAIRY CALVES. (Abstract) Jour. Dairy Sci. 19: 440-441.

(23) LONG, JOHN W., HUFFMAN, C.F. and DUNCAN, C.W. (1936). A STUDY OF THE VITAMIN D REQUIREMENTS OF CALVES WHEN NATURAL MILK FURNISHED THE SOLE SOURCE OF THE ANTIRACHITIC FACTOR. Milk Plant Monthly 25 (7): 30-36, 72, illus.

(24) McINTOSH, R.A. (1938). THE INDIGESTIONS OF RUMINANTS WITH SPECIAL REFERENCE TO TREATMENT. Cornell Vet. 28: 161-169.

(25) MADSEN, D.E. and NIELSEN, H.M. (1939). PARTURIENT HEMOGLOBINEMIA OF DAIRY cows. Amer. Vet. Med. Assoc. Jour. 94: 577-586, illus.

(26) ______and NIELSEN, H.M. (1940). THE RELATIONSHIP OF PARTURIENT HEMOGLOBINEMIA OF DAIRY COWS TO APROSPHOROSIS. North Amer. yet. 21: 81-89, illus.

(27) MADSEN, LOUIS L. (1939). FACTORS AFFECTING MAINTENANCE NUTRITION, FEED UTILIZATION AND HEALTH OF FARM ANIMALS., U.S. Dept. Agr. Yearbook (Food and Life) 1939: 431-449, illus.

(28) METZGIER, H.J. (1936). A CASE OF TETANY WITH HYPOMAGNESEMIA IN A DAIRY COW. Cornell Vet. 26: 353-356.

(29) MOORE, L.A. (1939). RELATIONSHIP BETWEEN CAROTENE, BLINDNESS DUE TO CONSTRICTION OF THE OPTIC NERVE, PAPILLARY EDEMA AND NYCTALOPIA IN CALVES. Jour. Nutr. 17: 443-459, illus.

(30) _______and HALLMAN, E.T. (1936). PRODUCTION OF WHITE SPOTTED KIDNEYS IN CALVES. (Abstract. of paper) Jour. Dairy Sci., 19: 434-435

(31) _______HALLMAN, E.T. and SHOLL, L.B. (1938). CARDIOVASCULAR AND OTHER LESIONS IN CALVES FED DIETS LOW IN MAGNESIUM. Arch. Path. 26: 820-838, illus.

(32) MOXON, ALVIN L. (1937). ALKALI DISEASE OR SELENIUM POISONING. S. Dak. Agr. Expt. Sta. Bul. 311, 91 pp., illus.

(33) NEAL,W.M. and AHMANN,C.F. (1937). COBALT AS AN ESSENTIAL ELEMENT IN ANIMAL NUTRITION. Science 86: 225-226, illus.

(34) _______and AHMANN, C.F. (1937). THE ESSENTIALITY OF COBALT IN BOVINE NUTRITION. Jour. Dairy Sci. 20: 741-753, illus.

(35) _______and BECKER, R.B. (1933). THE COMPOSITION OF FEEDSTUFFS IN RELATION TO NUTRITIONAL ANEMIA IN CATTLE. Jour. Agr. Res. 47: 249-255.

(36) NEWMAN, PAUL E. and SAVAGE, E.S. (1938). THE USE OF YEAST IN CALF MEALS AND PELLETS. Jour. Dairy Sci. 21: 161-167, illus.

(37) NEWSOM, I.E. (1938). URINARY CALCULI WITH SPECIAL REFERENCE TO CATTLE AND SHEEP. Amer. Vet. Med. Assoc. Jour. 92: 495-502.

(38) OLSON, T.M. (1940). BLOAT IN DAIRY CATTLE. Jour. Dairy Sci. 23: 343-353.

(39) OSLAND, H.B., MAYNARD, E.J. and MORTON, GEORGE E. (1936). COLARADO FATTENING RATIONS FOB CATTLE. Colo. Agr. Expt. Sta. Bur. 422, 120 pp., illus.

(40) PALMER, L.S., NELSON, J.W. and GULLICKSON, T.W. (1940). VITAMIN E POTENCY OF CERTAIN FOODSTUFFS. (Abstract of paper) Jour. Dairy Sci. 23: 571-572.

(41) PHILLIPS, PAUL H. (1940). DIRECTIONS FOR THE ASCORBIC ACID THERAPY OF SLOW-BREEDING BULLS. Amer. Vet. Med. Assoc. Jour. 97: 165-166.

(42) _______HART, E.B. and BOHST, G. (1934). CHRONIC TOXICOSIS IN DAIRY COWS DUE TO THE INGESTION OF FLUORINE. Wis. Agr. Expt. Sta. Res. But. 123. 30 pp., illus.

(43) _______LARDY, H.A. HEIZER, E.E. and RUPEL, I.W. (1940). SPERM STIMULATION IN THE BULL THROUGH THE SUBCUTANEOUS ADMINISTRATION OF ASCORBIC ACID. Jour. Dairy Sci. 23: 873-878.

(44) ______RUPEL, I.W., OLESON, J.J. and BOHSTEDT, G. (1938). THE EFFECTS OF AN A TYPICAL BLINDNESS-PRODUCING RATION UPON THE VITAMIN K AND C CONTENT OF CALF BLOOD. Amer. Soc. Anim. Prod. Proc. 31: 320-.327, illus.

(45) QUIN, A.H. (1939). SOME FACTORS INVOLVED IN THE DEFICIENCY DISEASES. Amer. Vet. Med. Assoc. Jour. 94: 621-626.

(46) REED, O.E. and HUFFMAN, C. F. (1930). THE RESULTS OF A FIVE-YEAR MINERAL FEEDING INVESTIGATION WITH DAIRY CATTLE. Mich. Agr. Expt. Sta. Tech. Bur. 105, 63 pp., illus.

(47) RIGGS, J.K. (1940). THE LENGTH OF TIME REQUIRED FOR DEPLETION OF VITAMIN A RESERVES IN RANGE CATTLE. Jour. Nutr. 20: 491-500.

(48) SHEELY, W.J. and SHEALY, A.L. (1940). BEEF PRODUCTION IN FLORIDA. Fla. UnIv. Agr. Ext. Bnl. 104, 35 pp., illus.

(49) SJOLLEMA, B. (1932). NUTRITIONAL AND METABOLIC DISORDERS IN CATTLE. Nutr. Abs. and Rev. 1: 621-632.

(50) SYKES, J.F. and ALFREDSON, B.V. (1940). STUDIES ON THE BOVINE ELECTROCARDIOGRAM. I. ELECTROCARDIOGRAPHIC CHANGES IN CALVES ON LOW POTASSIUM RATIONS. Sac. Expt. Biol. and Med. Proc. 43: 575-579, illus.

(51) THEILER, SIR ARNOLD and GREEN, HENRY H. (1932). APHOSPHOROSIS IN RUMINANTS. Nutr. Abs. and Rev. 1: 359-385.

(52) ______GREEN, HENRY HAMILTON and VILJOEN, PHILIP RUDOLPH (1915). CONTRIBUTION TO THE STUDY OF DEFICIENCY DISEASE, WITH SPECIAL REFERENCE TO THE LAMZIEKTE PROBLEM IN SOUTH AFRICA. Union So. Africa Dept. Agr., Dir. Vet. Res. Rpt. 3-4: 7-68.

INDEX

L

M

N